T0227230

Promoting Health and Wellness in the Geriatric Patient

Editor

DAVID A. SOTO-QUIJANO

PHYSICAL MEDICINE AND REHABILITATION CLINICS OF NORTH AMERICA

www.pmr.theclinics.com

Consulting Editor
SANTOS F. MARTINEZ

November 2017 • Volume 28 • Number 4

ELSEVIER

1600 John F. Kennedy Boulevard • Suite 1800 • Philadelphia, Pennsylvania, 19103-2899

http://www.theclinics.com

PHYSICAL MEDICINE AND REHABILITATION CLINICS OF NORTH AMERICA Volume 28, Number 4
November 2017 ISSN 1047-9651, ISBN 978-0-323-54897-7

Editor: Lauren Boyle
Developmental Editor: Meredith Madeira

Reprints. For copies of 100 or more of articles in this publication, please contact the Commercial Reprints Department, Elsevier Inc., 360 Park Avenue South, New York, NY 10010-1710. Tel.: 212-633-3874; Fax: 212-633-3820; E-mail: reprints@elsevier.com.

Physical Medicine and Rehabilitation Clinics of North America (ISSN 1047-9651) is published quarterly by Elsevier Inc., 360 Park Avenue South, New York, NY 10010-1710. Months of issue are February, May, August, and November. Business and Editorial Offices: 1600 John F. Kennedy Blvd., Suite 1800, Philadelphia, PA 19103-2899. Customer Service Office: 3251 Riverport Lane, Maryland Heights, MO 63043. Periodicals postage paid at New York, NY and additional mailing offices. Subscription price per year is $288.00 (US individuals), $560.00 (US institutions), $100.00 (US students), $210.00 (Canadian individuals), $737.00 (Canadian institutions), $210.00 (Canadian students), $210.00 (foreign individuals), $737.00 (foreign institutions), and $210.00 (foreign students). Foreign air speed delivery is included in all *Clinics* subscription prices. All prices are subject to change without notice. **POSTMASTER:** Send address changes to *Physical Medicine and Rehabilitation Clinics of North America*, Customer Service Office: Elsevier Health Sciences Division, Subscription Customer Service, 3251 Riverport Lane, Maryland Heights, MO 63043. **Customer Service: 1-800-654-2452 (US). From outside of the United States, call 314-447-8871. Fax: 314-447-8029. E-mail: JournalsCustomer Service-usa@elsevier.com (for print support); JournalsOnlineSupport-usa@elsevier.com (for online support).**

Physical Medicine and Rehabilitation Clinics of North America is indexed in *Excerpta Medica, MEDLINE/ PubMed (Index Medicus), Cinahl,* and *Cumulative Index to Nursing and Allied Health Literature.*

Contributors

CONSULTING EDITOR

SANTOS F. MARTINEZ, MD, MS
American Academy of Physical Medicine and Rehabilitation, Campbell Clinic
Orthopaedics, Department of Orthopaedics, The University of Tennessee, Memphis,
Tennessee

EDITOR

DAVID A. SOTO-QUIJANO, MD, FAAPMR
Director, Physical Medicine and Rehabilitation Residency Program, VA Caribbean
Healthcare System, San Juan, Puerto Rico

AUTHORS

JESSICA L. AU, MD
Department of Rehabilitation Medicine, NewYork Presbyterian Hospital, Harkness
Pavilion, Hudson Spine & Pain Medicine, New York, New York

DAVID BEATON-COMULADA, MD
Research Fellow, Department of Orthopaedic Surgery, School of Medicine, University of
Puerto Rico, San Juan, Puerto Rico

MELISSA BERNSTEIN, PhD, RD, LD, FAND
Assistant Professor, Department of Nutrition, Chicago Medical School, Rosalind Franklin
University of Medicine and Science, North Chicago, Illinois

BRENDA CASTILLO, MD
Chief Resident, Department of Physical Medicine and Rehabilitation, VA Caribbean
Healthcare System, San Juan, Puerto Rico

JOHN C. CIANCA, MD
Adjunct Associate Professor of Physical Medicine and Rehabilitation, Baylor College of
Medicine, University of Texas Health Science Center, Owner, Human Performance
Center, Medical Director, Houston Marathon Committee, Houston, Texas

MARICARMEN CRUZ-JIMENEZ, MD
Attending Physician, Physical Medicine and Rehabilitation, VA Caribbean Healthcare
System, Assistant Professor, Physical Medicine and Rehabilitation, University of Puerto
Rico, San Juan, Puerto Rico

RAMON CUEVAS-TRISAN, MD
Chief, Physical Medicine and Rehabilitation Service, West Palm Beach VA Medical Center,
University of Miami Miller School of Medicine, Nova Southeastern University College of
Osteopathic Medicine, West Palm Beach, Florida

JOEL E. FRONTERA, MD
Assistant Professor, Residency Program Director, Vice-Chair for Education, Department of Physical Medicine and Rehabilitation, McGovern Medical School, The University of Texas Health Science Center at Houston, Houston, Texas

WALTER R. FRONTERA, MD, PhD
Professor, Departments of Physical Medicine, Rehabilitation, and Sports Medicine and Physiology, School of Medicine, University of Puerto Rico, San Juan, Puerto Rico

JUAN GALLOZA, MD
Assistant Professor, Department of Physical Medicine and Rehabilitation, McGovern Medical School, The University of Texas Health Science Center at Houston, TIRR Memorial Hermann, Houston, Texas

EKUA GILBERT-BAFFOE, MD
Department of Physical Medicine and Rehabilitation, Baylor College of Medicine, Houston, Texas

PRATHAP JAYARAM, MD
Assistant Professor, Physical Medicine and Rehabilitation and Orthopedic Surgery, Director of Regenerative Sports Medicine, Baylor College of Medicine, Houston, Texas

MANUEL F. MAS, MD
Assistant Professor, Department of Physical Medicine and Rehabilitation, McGovern Medical School, The University of Texas Health Science Center at Houston, TIRR Memorial Hermann, Houston, Texas

AMY MATHEWS, MD
Department of Physical Medicine and Rehabilitation, Baylor College of Medicine, Houston, Texas

WILLIAM MICHEO, MD
Professor and Chair, Sports Medicine Fellowship Director, Department of Physical Medicine, Rehabilitation and Sports Medicine, School of Medicine, University of Puerto Rico, San Juan, Puerto Rico

PATRICK MOLLETT, DO
Resident Physician, Department of Physical Medicine and Rehabilitation, McGovern Medical School, The University of Texas Health Science Center at Houston, Houston, Texas

JENNIFER P. MOODY, MD
Department of Rehabilitation Medicine, NewYork Presbyterian Hospital, Harkness Pavilion, New York, New York

ANTONIO OTERO-LÓPEZ, MD, FAAOS
Program Director, Department of Orthopaedic Surgery, School of Medicine, University of Puerto Rico, San Juan, Puerto Rico

JESUEL PADRO-GUZMAN, MD
Department of Neurology, Memorial Sloan Kettering Cancer Center, Division of Rehabilitation Medicine, Weill Cornell Medicine, New York, New York

JOSE LUIS PESANTE-PINTO, MD
Professor, Ambulatory Medicine Coordinator, Family Medicine Department, Universidad Central del Caribe School of Medicine, Bayamon, Puerto Rico

CARLOS E. RIVERA-TAVAREZ, MD
Staff Physician, Campbell Clinic Orthopedics, Memphis, Tennessee

RICARDO M. RODRIGUEZ, PhD
Clinical Psychologist, Physical Medicine and Rehabilitation Service, VA Caribbean Healthcare System, San Juan, Puerto Rico

DAVID A. SOTO-QUIJANO, MD, FAAPMR
Director, Physical Medicine and Rehabilitation Residency Program, VA Caribbean Healthcare System, San Juan, Puerto Rico

Contents

Older adults 65 years of age and older compose a great portion of the US population. Physiologic changes of aging that limit function and general quality of life occur at a faster rate as we get older. There is high-quality evidence that exercise activity has many favorable benefits for older adults. The ideal exercise program in older adults should include aerobic, resistance, flexibility, and balance training. The exercise recommendations should be individually tailored to the abilities, precautions, and goals of each person. They also should be of sufficient intensity, volume, and duration to achieve maximal benefits.

Aging is an inevitable multifactorial process. Advances in health care and technology have led to an increase on expected life span that can reach an average of 90 years in the next few decades. Lifestyle changes that include activity, nutrition, stress management, and alternative low-impact exercises like yoga and tai chi can help us modify some of these age-related changes and lead to an increase in the health span and quality of life of the older adults.

The deterioration of physical and mental capabilities is inevitable with aging. Some hereditary factors cannot be changed, but other external factors can be manipulated to provide our body with better weapons to improve quality of life as we age. Different cellular pathways leading to cell deterioration and aging usually act through excessive oxidative damage and chronic inflammation. Suppression of inflammation is the most important driver of successful longevity and increases in importance with advancing age. Modifying caloric intake, amount and type of food, and maintaining an active lifestyle can decrease the risk of most common chronic diseases of aging.

Geriatric patients present multiple age-related challenges and needs that must be taken into account during the rehabilitation process to achieve expected goals. This article examines the importance of identifying and managing psychosocial issues commonly observed in older adults and presents strategies to optimize their rehabilitation process. Depression, anxiety, fear of falling, adjustment issues, neurocognitive disorders, and caregiver support are discussed as a selection of factors that are relevant for geriatric patients undergoing rehabilitation. An argument is made for the importance of comprehensive geriatric assessment in older adults to identify salient issues that may impact rehabilitation and quality of life.

Aging is one of the important challenges of modern society. Advanced adult age is associated with changes in many physiologic systems. Of particular interest is the musculoskeletal system because it directly contributes to mobility and functional independence. Skeletal muscle mass and strength decline with age. These changes are mostly due to a reduction in the number of muscle fibers and cellular and molecular changes that reduce the force-generation process. Bone mass and architecture are compromised and may result in fractures. Tendons and ligaments undergo significant biochemical alterations that directly compromise their biomechanical function.

There are normal physiologic changes that occur as people age. Gait and mobility are altered with aging, and these changes are a combination of alterations in the gait pattern and in the function of organs. Changes in gait are associated with functional decline, less independence, and impaired quality of life. Reduced walking speed is the most consistent age-related change, but there are other contributors to an altered gait: impaired balance and stability, lower extremity strength, and the fear of falling.

Falls in the elderly are an increasing problem causing a high degree of morbidity, mortality, and use of health care services. Identification of risk factors through medical assessment supports the provision of appropriate interventions that reduce rates of falling. Evaluation and intervention strategies are generally challenging because of the complex and multifactorial nature of falls. The clinician should consider screening for falls an important part of the functional evaluation in older adults. Several potential interventions have proven helpful as preventive strategies. Optimal approaches involve interdisciplinary collaboration in assessment and interventions, particularly exercise, attention to coexisting medical conditions, and reduction of environmental hazards.

Elderly people have several characteristics that make them unique. They have environmental and demographic factors, such as age, sex, socioeconomic level, and schooling, which contribute to these differences being accentuated. As one ages, these various organic and systemic features are accentuated. The pace varies between people, and organs and systems suffer from several normal and adverse changes that make them more or less susceptible to diseases and injuries, and medications are responsible for many of these threats. This article raises awareness about these changes.

Older adults are particularly vulnerable to compromised nutritional status. With advancing age, the consumption of a high-quality, nutritionally dense diet is increasingly essential to optimize health and well-being. Proportionally, macronutrient needs for older adults are similar to younger adults; however, overall calorie requirements tend to decline with age. Unique factors influencing food intake should be considered and individualized guidance should be designed to help overcome medical, physical, and social barriers to a healthy diet. The goal for nutrition intervention should ultimately be to promote health and quality of life across the continuum of the aging process.

Clinicians should discuss common health issues of the older population and how medical problems affect their sports performance. Patients with chronic conditions, such as hypertension and diabetes mellitus, benefit from participation in sports. However, special care should be taken to keep the patient healthy and minimize effects of these conditions and their treatments in athletic performance. Another important consideration in the older athlete is fluid ingestion and the increased risk of dehydration. There is evidence that physical exercise reduces pain in osteoarthritis and enhances physical function of affected joints. Older athletes often use multiple medications and dietary supplements. Clinicians should educate patients about possible effects of medications in sports performance.

Regenerative medicine has gained increasing popularity in its clinical applications, particularly in the field of musculoskeletal medicine.

Regenerative medicine, a broad term, can be thought of as a particular medical strategy that strives to rebuild and restore diseased tissue to normal physiologic tissue baseline. Simply put, regenerative strategies augment the body's innate physiology to heal pathologic processes. This article focuses on specific regenerative strategies and the uses of them for common pathologies in the aging adult, including platelet-rich plasma, mesenchymal stem cells, viscosupplementation, and prolotherapy.

There is an increase in the aging population that has led to a surge of reported cases of osteoarthritis and a greater demand for lower extremity arthroplasty. This article aims to review the current treatment options and expectations when considering lower extremity arthroplasty in the elderly patient with an emphasis on the following subjects: updated clinical guidelines for the management of osteoarthritis in the lower extremity, comorbidities and risk factors in the surgical patient, preoperative evaluation and optimization of the surgical patient, surgical approach and implant selection, and rehabilitation and life after lower extremity arthroplasty.

Physiatrists taking care of the geriatric patient with cancer should be able to manage an array of conditions that might present from diagnosis throughout completion of treatments and beyond. The elderly cancer population is at greater risk of functional impairments. The physician should anticipate changes in clinical status and must adjust rehabilitation goals accordingly. Treatment options and rehabilitation goals should be tailored to help maximize quality of life in these patients.

The 2016 National Spinal Cord Injury Statistical Center's *Spinal Cord Injury* (SCI) *Facts and Figures* reports approximately 17,000 new cases yearly, approximately 54 cases per million. The past 40 years has brought a significant change in patterns of injury. The average age has increased from 29 years in the 1970s to approximately 42 years currently; it is believed it has plateaued. Aging persons with SCI may have a higher risk of developing other medical complications. Studies report a perceived improvement in quality of life among persons with SCI with age, influenced by psychological, medical, and environmental factors.

The incidence of traumatic brain injury (TBI) in older adults is increasing. As the expected life expectancy increases, there is a heightened need for comprehensive rehabilitation for this population. Elderly patients with TBI benefit from rehabilitation interventions at all stages of injury and can achieve functional gains during acute inpatient rehabilitation. Clinicians should be vigilant of unique characteristics of this population during inpatient rehabilitation, including vulnerability to polypharmacy, posttraumatic hydrocephalus, neuropsychiatric sequelae, sleep disturbances, and sensory deficits. Long-term care should include fall prevention, assessment of cognitive deficits, aerobic activity, community reintegration, and caretaker support. Life expectancy is reduced after TBI.

PHYSICAL MEDICINE AND REHABILITATION CLINICS OF NORTH AMERICA

FORTHCOMING ISSUES

February 2018
Interventional Spine Procedures
Carlos E. Rivera, *Editor*

May 2018
Para Sports Medicine
Yetsa A. Tuakli-Wosornu and
Wayne Derman, *Editors*

August 2018
Muscle Over-activity in Upper Motor Neuron Syndrome: Assessment and Problem Solving for Complex Cases
Miriam Segal, *Editor*

RECENT ISSUES

August 2017
Pelvic Pain
Kelly M. Scott, *Editor*

May 2017
Traumatic Brain Injury Rehabilitation
Blessen C. Eapen and David X. Cifu, *Editors*

February 2017
Adjunctive Rehabilitation Approaches to Oncology
Andrea L. Cheville, *Editor*

RELATED INTEREST

Clinics in Geriatric Medicine, November 2016 (Vol. 32, Issue 4)
Geriatric Pain Management
M. Carrington Reid, *Editor*

VISIT THE CLINICS ONLINE!
Access your subscription at:
www.theclinics.com

Foreword

As a general rule, getting old beats the alternative every time. I have lived 75 years with a developmental disability and have practiced medicine for 50 years, and I ought to know.

Treating geriatric patients who have disabilities is not the same thing as treating geriatric patients and treating patients with disabilities. Treating elderly patients who have disabilities requires that we be alert for signs that might not be significant in other populations.

A 54-year-old man who had cerebral palsy and was employed by the state came to the clinic complaining that his walking was becoming worse. The physicians who examined him ordered blood work, found nothing significant, and sent him home. Three months later, he returned to the clinic, saying that his walking had continued to deteriorate. He was told that he probably had a virus and was again sent home. Three months after that, he returned, saying that not only his walking was much worse but now he was also experiencing weakness in his arms.

At this point a rehabilitation consult was requested, and the physiatrist ordered an MRI, which showed a cervical cord myelopathy due to a spinal cord compression.

Had the patient been 80 years old, the diagnosis might have been suspected at his first visit, but at 54, he was too young to have a spinal myelopathy. The fact of his cerebral palsy should have modified the physicians' understanding of his complaint.

Physical presentations can be confusing to nonspecialists, but other problems in older patients who have disabilities require a more subtle approach.

In the early 1970s, I enjoyed a practice involving patients with all kinds of disabilities. My special interest was in the psychological development of adolescents with disabilities. My boss, Dr Dorothea Glass, chair of PM&R at Temple, asked me to go to the Philadelphia Geriatric Center and create a program for elderly people with disabilities. I decided to bring the pediatric therapists I had been working with along with me to the geriatric program.

The therapists while working with the teenage rehabilitation patients had found them to be much more cooperative and willing to work hard when they felt they had some control over their rehabilitation program. There are many ways to work the same muscle groups, so instead of prescribing what the patients were to do, the therapists made the patients part of the team, offering them choices as to how they would work their bodies. Given choices, the adolescents became invested in their own success, and their excellent results reflected their enthusiasm.

The therapists approached the geriatric patients in the same way, involving them in the creation of their own programs of exercise, with the same results. Allowed to choose, the patients felt empowered and more responsible for achieving their goals, resulting in superior outcomes.

We found that speech and OT were more palatable to our geriatric rehabilitation patients if we offered these therapies in a group setting. The stronger patients pushed the weaker to try harder, to move toward success for the group.

Phys Med Rehabil Clin N Am 28 (2017) xiii–xvii
http://dx.doi.org/10.1016/j.pmr.2017.09.002
1047-9651/17/© 2017 Published by Elsevier Inc.

pmr.theclinics.com

Over the five years I was involved with the program, about 100 residential patients moved through the rehabilitation program. Ordinarily, patients over time would move to the next, higher, level of care, but the patients we treated in a group moved back to a previous level of care. Thirty-seven of the patients came for outpatient therapy with the expectation that they, too, would be moving into residential care, but these patients all returned to their homes.

The average age of the patients treated in a group was 82. At the time, they were not expected to live many more years, and there were questions about how much effort should be put their rehabilitation. Now we know that a person who lives to age 82 can expect to live about seven years longer.

In 1980, I presided over the first major conference on geriatric rehabilitation, and I decided to revisit my patients from 1976. I found that only two of the original 37 patients had died during the intervening years, and the rest of them were still living—at home.

Geriatric patients may be hesitant to talk to younger physicians about sensitive topics, so it is up to us to broach areas of concern that too often are overlooked in the treatment of older rehab patients.

Sex can be very difficult for older patients to bring up during a visit, and too often the assumption is made that there is no such thing as geriatric sexual activity. It is important to talk with patients about their sex lives and to include screening for sexually transmitted diseases when appropriate, particularly since disabilities and medications may disguise symptoms of STDs.

During the 1940s and 1950s, thousands of children with disabilities were institutionalized. These children are older adults now, and there is a good chance that some of the geriatric rehabilitation patients we treat come from this population. We are aware now that sexual abuse of institutionalized children was rampant, and particularly common with children who are disabled. Awareness of the possibility that a patient was sexually abused as a child should help guide us in diagnosis: persistent abdominal pain, increased spasticity, or autonomic dysreflexia may be due to an untreated STD or sexual injury.[1]

Patients with disabilities are at greatly increased risk of elder abuse, another area where a clinician's willingness to ask about symptoms that may not be obvious on physical examination is crucial. Recent statistics support greater concern for disabled adult patients: Thirty-three percent of adult women with disabilities report experiencing interpersonal violence, versus 21% of institutionalized women who are not disabled.[2]

In one study, 55% of men reported physical abuse after becoming disabled, nearly 12% of them by a personal assistance provider.[3]

A comprehensive review of the literature from 2000 to 2010 showed violence of all types against adult women with disabilities ranged from 36% to 90%. Reported abuse against men with disabilities revealed similar percentages.[4]

The US Centers for Disease Control and Prevention reported that incidences of sexual violence against women with disabilities range from 51% to 79%, depending on the state. Another study found that 92% of women with disabilities suffered blows to the head, with 40% losing consciousness during the attack.[5–8]

Finances may be as difficult as sexual matters for older patients to bring up during an examination. People with disabilities earn less per hour and work fewer hours per week than the nondisabled population. The average household income of people with disabilities is 75% lower than that of people who do not have disabilities.

One-third of widowed American women over age 65 and with a disability do not have enough money to buy food. If they are women of color, that number goes to 49.5%. This is a national disgrace!

Given that food insecurity can have immense effects on health, screening should be done in this population to rule out nutritional issues related to inadequate finances. The choice between paying for medicine and paying for food is not just a cliché—it is a reality we must deal with in our patients. I believe sufficient food and medical care are civil rights and must be protected as such.

Patients who need assistance with activities of daily living must deal with caregivers who may or may not be family members. Caregivers can fall into two categories: those who help the patient do what the patient wants done, and those who do for the patient what the caregiver feels should be done. People with disabilities who rely on caregivers can feel frustrated and miserable if the caregiver does not respect the patient enough to function as an amanuensis rather than a supervisor, particularly if the patient is competent. Respect for the patient defines the caregiver's role, and a caregiver who does not respect the patient's wishes should not be tolerated.

Preserving mobility should be a prime goal in caring for older patients with disabilities. Walking, going up and down stairs, and/or using a rowing or Nu-step machine should be part of the patient's daily routine. The NIH has recommended tai chi and qi gong, ancient practices of gentle movement, as ideal exercises for older people.[9] The more mobile a patient can remain, the less she is likely to be subjected to someone else's control.

Helping a patient who has dementia remain at home for as long as possible can be challenging to the family, but there are fairly simple and inexpensive steps that can be taken to preserve the patient's dignity and safety. Most dementia patients are moved out of the family home because of incontinence of bladder and bowel. Making the toilet easier for the patient to locate and use can reduce incidents of incontinence. The patient's personal items, such as a towel, toothbrush, comb, and so forth, should be a different, bright color from those of the rest of the family; the toilet seat should be of a contrasting color to the color of the rest of the bathroom—a white bathroom should have a black toilet seat, for example—and a light and radio should be left on in the bathroom the patient uses, both to make it easier to find and to remind the patient to use it. Door alarms throughout the house will help keep the patient safe and reassure family members. These steps are practical, but perhaps more important, they can help preserve the patient's dignity.

A patient with Alzheimer was living at home, doing well, until one day she could not be found in the house. Wandering away is an all-too-frequent risk of dementia, one that can lead to death from exposure, drowning, or being struck by a car.

The patient's relieved family found her on the sidewalk, looking for the bus stop. She wanted to go shopping.

This family's loving and creative solution to the problem had an impact beyond their own relative. They built a "bus stop" just outside their house, with a shelter and bench. The patient could go outside and wait for the bus, happily anticipating her shopping trip and feeling independent that she could do this on her own. After a while, her family would lead her back into the house. One day, they noticed that there were two people sitting at the bus stop—it had become a meeting place for the neighborhood, a place where a person with Alzheimer could have a casual conversation with her neighbors.

The most important rotation of my medical training was Internal Medicine. I was assigned to a huge room in Bellevue Hospital, a room filled with 40 beds and attended by a first-year resident and two interns. The resident was a Vietnam Vet who couldn't understand why someone like me had been accepted to medical school, and who made it his mission to make my life as miserable as possible. He was successful.

One of my patients was an 80-year-old woman with congestive heart failure. I performed her history and physical examination, and then I needed to draw blood for her lab work. The lady was reluctant to allow me to do this, and she appealed to the intern, who told her very kindly that I was her doctor and it was an important part of my training to draw her blood.

She eventually, reluctantly, agreed. I drew the blood without any problem. It was an important moment for both of us.

I became very fond of this lady and would often stop by to visit with her. One day, I was sitting on her bed, holding her hand while we talked, and the resident came by. He flew into a rage, screaming loud enough for all forty patients and the other interns to hear that my behavior was totally inappropriate and that I was never going to be a doctor. I left, totally demoralized. Much later I realized that the problem was his, not mine.

I had grown up in a multigenerational household; my grandparents lived with my parents and me almost from the day I was born. I was lucky in many ways to have known older people intimately for my entire childhood. I treasure happy memories to this day of eating hard-boiled eggs (with lots of butter!) upstairs in my grandmother's kitchen and of my grandfather doing pushups with my sister and me sitting, giggling, on his back.

To me, it was only natural to sit with the old lady at Bellevue, holding her hand and talking. Our childhood experiences shape us all, and it is important to draw on the lessons we learned as children to help us see our elderly patients today not as off-putting strangers, but as part of our human family.

How a society treats the most vulnerable of its population is a measure of its strength. A society that devalues what it defines as weakness will not survive.

In ancient times, the mission of the warrior class in Athens was to protect and care for the weak; in Sparta, the weak were culled to make the warrior class strong.

Sparta no longer exists.

The most rapidly growing segments of our population are

1. People over 80
2. People over 65
3. People with disabilities

One day I was driving home from work, and I noticed an old man on the sidewalk. Something told me he was in trouble, and I pulled over and asked him if he needed help. "I'm lost," he told me. He was trying to get home. He gave me his address; he was a couple of blocks over from where he needed to be. I offered him a ride, and I drove him to his house.

Paying attention to nonverbal cues—body language, facial expression—can help in diagnosing older patients, especially patients who may have trouble describing just what is wrong. Ignoring our common instinct to offer unsolicited help can help mask symptoms.

For forty years, I've owned a shore house. When I was young, I could walk down the beach to swim in the ocean. Over time, it became difficult for me to get down to the water. I got a recumbent tricycle I could ride up and down the boardwalk, but I was unable to get into the sand and play with my grandchildren. I had to sit alone on the boardwalk and watch my family enjoy the ocean. A couple of years ago I found out about the Magic Mobility X8, a vehicle that can drive me over the sand, down to the beach with my grandchildren. Check me out on YouTube at Magic Mobility Extreme X-8: Meet Dr. Strax. Technology that results in better medical treatment is of course very important, but technology that helps preserve the dignity of the patient while enhancing his ability to be an active part of his family—and of society—is equally important.

Thomas E. Strax, MD
1003 Easton Road
Willow Grove, PA 19090, USA

Martha Sprowles, BA
945 Langhorne Yardley Road
Langhorne, PA 19047, USA

E-mail addresses:
tstrax@icloud.com (T.E. Strax)
m_sprowles@verizon.net (M. Sprowles)

REFERENCES

1. Weiner SL. Sexually transmitted infections in women with disabilities: diagnosis, treatment and prevention: a review. Sex Transm Dis 2000;27:272–7.
2. Barrett KA, O'Day B, Roche A, et al. Intimate partner violence, health status, and health care access among women with disabilities. Womens Health Issues 2009;19(2):94–100.
3. Powers L, Saxton M, Curry M, et al. End the silence: a survey of abuse against men with disabilities. J Rehabil 2008;74(4):41–53.
4. Hughes R, Lund E, Gabrielli J, et al. Prevalence of interpersonal violence against community-living adults with disabilities: a literature review. Rehabil Psychol 2011;56(4):302–19.
5. Centers for Disease Control and Prevention. Sexual violence against people with disabilities. 2002. Available at: http://www.cdc.gov/ncicp/factsheets. Accessed September 16, 2017.
6. Basile KC, Saltzman LE. Sexual violence surveillance: uniform definitions and recommended data elements. Version 1.0. Atlanta (GA): National Center for Injury Prevention and Control, Centers for Disease Control and Prevention; 2002.
7. Abramson WH. California Coalition Against Sexual Assault (serving survivors of sexual assault with disabilities). Sacramento (CA): CALCASA; 2001.
8. Weinstein DD, Martin PR. Neurologic disorders and head injuries in substance abuse in the mentally and physically disabled. In: Hubbard JR, Martin PR, editors. Substance abuse in the mentally and physically disabled. New York: Marcel Dekker; 2001. p. 277–305.
9. Available at: https://nccih.nih.gov/health/taichi/introduction.htm#hed1. Accessed September 16, 2017.

Foreword

Aging with Grace, Dignity, and Courage: A Mission for Physical Medicine and Rehabilitation

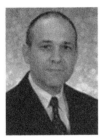

Santos F. Martinez, MD, MS
Consulting Editor

Our perspectives and priorities in life change as we age and take care of those aging. Although the physical medicine and rehabilitation (PMR) specialty has a special privilege and sensitivity caring for those challenged by a spectrum of physical and neurocognitive limitations, it could not be expressed better than by our exemplary physician, educator, and leader in PMR, Dr Strax. His foreword provides us with decades of wisdom both as a physician and one living with his disability.

I thank Dr Soto-Quijano for giving us an amalgam of authors providing transitional aging approaches to optimize one's quality of life whether disabled or not. The collection of topics also reflects an evolvement in physical medicine and rehabilitation with information that is useful for those treating inpatients or purely outpatients. Many in our field are becoming more visible outside of the traditional rehab setting with promotion of factors that contribute to wellness. We certainly do not intend to neglect our heritage but complement traditional approaches to meet future needs of our population. We need to be at the forefront insuring that our population is empowered with the tools to facilitate and optimize function. We need to better refine screening tools for assessing declines (neurocognitive, vision, hearing, cardiopulmonary, strength, balance, nutrition, psychosocial, and so forth) again whether those be attributed solely to aging or combined with other disabilities. As in many fields, the transition from crisis management and completion of rehabilitation to more proactive preventive approaches is natural and will certainly be a great

Phys Med Rehabil Clin N Am 28 (2017) xix–xx
http://dx.doi.org/10.1016/j.pmr.2017.09.003
1047-9651/17/© 2017 Published by Elsevier Inc.

complement to our clinical practice. I thank all the authors for their hard work for this issue.

Santos F. Martinez, MD, MS
American Academy of Physical Medicine
and Rehabilitation
Campbell Clinic Orthopaedics
Department of Orthopaedics
University of Tennessee
Memphis, TN 38104, USA

E-mail address:
smartinez@campbellclinic.com

Preface

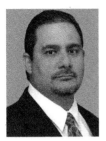

David A. Soto-Quijano, MD, FAAPMR
Editor

Twenty years ago, during my early years as a physical medicine and rehabilitation resident, evaluating subjects over 80 years of age in the outpatient clinics was a rare occurrence. Seeing patients over 90 years was an event, often discussed during lunchtime with amazement. The few patients of this age group that we treated then were usually accompanied by their relatives, using assistive devices and mostly asking for assistive equipment and palliative care. Nowadays to take care of patients over 80 years is not rare and seeing individuals over 90 is increasingly common. Some of these patients come to us on their own, driving their own cars and asking for help to continue their very fulfilling, independent lives. As physiatrists and promoters of an active lifestyle, it is particularly rewarding to take care of older patients that still play golf, ride their bikes, swim, and exercise regularly during the so-called golden years.

Unfortunately, that is not the reality of most people of old age. Medical care advances and public health initiatives have allowed more people to live longer lives. But the quality of life of many of these individuals is far from optimal. With the aging of the population, the need of more ventures to improve the life of our older individuals will increase greatly. The World Health Organization invites us to create an age-friendly society.[1] As physiatrists, we possess a great number of tools that could be instrumental in this transformation into a world that provides opportunities and fulfills the needs of our older population. It could also be important to remember that with good health care and maybe a little luck, we will all become part of that older age group and will eventually benefit directly from all the changes that we are proposing today.

In this issue of *Physical Medicine and Rehabilitation Clinics of North America*, we want to focus on strategies that can promote health and wellness in geriatric patients. An assessment of the medical needs of the older competitive athletes and the benefits of exercise in this age group, including innovative modalities like dance, tai-chi, and yoga, remind us of the importance of physical activity. For a better understanding of the needs of this population, we review the changes expected in the musculoskeletal system and the nutritional needs as we age. We also discuss common problems of the elderly that can create a barrier to a better life, including geriatric syndromes, polypharmacy, balance problems, fall risks, mobility, and alterations in gait.

Phys Med Rehabil Clin N Am 28 (2017) xxi–xxii
http://dx.doi.org/10.1016/j.pmr.2017.09.001
1047-9651/17/© 2017 Published by Elsevier Inc.

pmr.theclinics.com

As physiatrists, we deal with special populations that are also tending to live longer. The particular medical needs and issues of older patients after traumatic brain injury, spinal cord injury, and cancer are reviewed by physiatrists who specialize in these subjects. Common psychosocial issues in the geriatric population and its effect in rehabilitation are other important topics worth reviewing as they can affect our rehabilitation interventions. We also include an update of osteoarthritis and other common musculoskeletal disorders, including the possible role of regenerative injections in their treatment. Finally, we examine a difficult question that is increasingly occupying the minds of scientists: Can we increase our health span?

The task of promoting health and wellness in the elderly is monumental and will take a big effort from the medical community and society in general. It is our goal that through this issue we could help our field to meet this huge challenge. We hope that this information will be helpful in managing our older patients more effectively. But we also hope that it can create awareness among our colleagues that by improving the quality of life of this population we will be building a better future for our society.

David A. Soto-Quijano, MD, FAAPMR
Physical Medicine and Rehabilitation
Residency Program
VA Caribbean Healthcare System
San Juan, Puerto Rico

E-mail address:
David.soto-quijano@va.gov

REFERENCE

1. World Report on Ageing and Health 2015. http://apps.who.int/iris/bitstream/10665/186463/1/9789240694811_eng.pdf.

Benefits of Exercise in the Older Population

Juan Galloza, MD[a], Brenda Castillo, MD[b], William Micheo, MD[c],*

KEYWORDS

- Exercise • Physical activity • Older adults • Elderly • Aerobic • Resistance
- Flexibility • Balance

KEY POINTS

- The older adult population has been on an increasing trend in the past years and is expected to continue increasing over the next 20 years.
- There are several physiologic changes associated with aging that will cause a progressive decline in function.
- Exercise activity has been well established as a preventive and treatment strategy to counteract the detrimental changes of aging.
- An appropriate exercise program should include a combination of aerobic, resistance, flexibility, and balance exercises.
- The exercise recommendations should be individually tailored to the abilities, precautions, and goals of each person.

INTRODUCTION

Older adults 65 years of age and older compose 13% of the US population according to the US Census of 2010, an increase of 15% when compared with the previous census of the year 2000. This trend is expected to continue and will result in a 20% of the total population by the year 2030 being considered old.[1,2] Physiologic changes of aging that limit function and general quality of life (QOL), occur at a faster rate as we get older.[3] Sedentary behavior also increases with age making older adults the most sedentary population, with 65% to 80% of their waking time spent sitting.[4] This lack of physical activity has negative effects on cardio-metabolic health, muscle-tendon

Disclosure: The authors have nothing to disclose.
[a] Department of Physical Medicine and Rehabilitation, McGovern Medical School, The University of Texas Health Science Center at Houston, TIRR Memorial Hermann, 1333 Moursund Street, Houston, TX 770030, USA; [b] Department of Physical Medicine and Rehabilitation, VA Caribbean Healthcare System, 10, Calle Casia, San Juan, PR 00921, USA; [c] Department of Physical Medicine, Rehabilitation and Sports Medicine, School of Medicine, University of Puerto Rico, Office A-204, PO Box 365067, San Juan, PR 00926, USA
* Corresponding author.
E-mail address: william.micheo@upr.edu

Phys Med Rehabil Clin N Am 28 (2017) 659–669
http://dx.doi.org/10.1016/j.pmr.2017.06.001

health, functional fitness, physical independence, body composition, and all-cause mortality. Conversely, exercise has been well established as a preventive strategy as well as a medical intervention to counteract the detrimental effects of aging.[5]

Exercise programs in older adults should include aerobic, resistance, flexibility, and balance training. Each individual type of exercise may benefit different health-related factors, but the combination of all is essential for an effective exercise program in the older adult population.

AEROBIC/ENDURANCE
Basic Concepts

Aerobic capacity measured by maximum oxygen consumption (Vo_{2max}) shows a steady decline with age, as much as 10% per decade after 25 years of age. This decline is mainly due to decreased cardiac output that is caused by an increased peripheral circulatory resistance.[6] Other related factors, such as stroke volume, maximal heart rate, total plasma volume, and thirst sensation, also decrease with age.[7]

Aerobic exercise training (AET) refers to exercises in which the large muscles of the body move in a rhythmic manner for sustained periods of time. Examples of exercise activities with aerobic components are walking, running, stair climbing, cycling, swimming, or rowing. These types of exercises use energy through oxidative metabolism, which is the most important pathway for energy production during prolonged exercise activity.[8]

What is the Evidence?

The effects of AET can be assessed by measuring aerobic capacity, changes in heart rate and blood pressure, changes in glucose and lipid metabolism, among others. There is high-quality evidence that AET of moderate-high intensity significantly improves Vo_{2max} in older adults.[9] The improvements observed are comparable with those that occur in younger adults, except in adults older than 75 years when the rate of improvement is less. There is also evidence that AET programs, more so in high intensity than moderate intensity, enhance glycemic control. Improvements in postprandial lipid metabolism has also been evidenced independent of dietary modification.[9] Villareal and colleagues[10] showed that an exercise program including AET as well as other forms of exercise caused significant improvements in performance testing and other frailty parameters, including Vo_{2max} and Functional Status Questionnaire. The case is not the same for other parameters like body weight/composition and bone health, whereby the evidence shows that changes in decreased total body fat, increased fat-free mass, and increased bone mineral density have been modest.

Benefits in Chronic Disease

AET programs have well-established benefits for decreasing cardiovascular risk factors. They induce favorable adaptations to traditional risk factors, including lower heart rate at rest and during submaximal exercise, smaller increases in blood pressure, increase in glucose transporter content in muscle, improved whole-body insulin action, and a reduction in plasma lipid concentrations.[9] The beneficial effects of AET are not only related to the more traditional risk factors but also aerobic exercise interventions in older adults have shown improvements in large elastic arterial stiffness and vascular endothelial function.[6,11]

Exercise Recommendations

Initially the aerobic exercise program for an older adult should start with a low level of activity and ideally progress to moderate activity (50%–60% of pretraining Vo_{2max}).

The average moderate activity level for most older adults is 2.5 to 5.5 metabolic equivalents, which is the same as walking at a 2.0 to 4.5 miles per hour (mph) pace or cycling at 10 mph or less.[2] An easier recommendation for the individual to follow is to exercise at the maximal intensity while still being able to easily maintain conversation. In order to achieve a safe and adequate level of effort, it is recommended for older adults to start in a supervised exercise program. Aerobic exercise should be performed for 3 days or more per week for a total of 30 minutes with warm-up and cool-down periods of 5 to 10 minutes of low-intensity activity. The benefits of AET are observed with programs lasting more than 4 months, and even greater benefits are observed with AET programs lasting more than 6 months.[2,5,9] It is recommended that cycling, elliptical walker, and aquatic aerobic exercises should be considered as an alternative for older adults with conditions that may limit weight-bearing activity. Stationary recumbent cycling may be considered as an option for older adults with low-back pain or poor balance.

RESISTANCE/STRENGTHENING
Basic Concepts

Sarcopenia in the elderly population has been associated with reduced functionality, frailty, and disability. The progressive decline in muscle mass and strength accelerates after 65 years of age; by 80 years of age, up to 50% of peak skeletal muscle mass can be lost. This normal aging phenomenon has been related to lack of physical activity, loss of muscle fibers, protein synthesis, and mitochondrial function.[3,12]

Strengthening or resistance exercise training (RET) has been a known effective method to counteract the age-related changes of sarcopenia by improving muscle mass, strength, and function.[13–15] RET includes static (isometric) and dynamic muscle contractions. Static or isometric contractions produce force without joint movement or changes in muscle length. They are useful in older individuals when movement of the joint is restricted because of pain or injury. Dynamic contractions can be further divided into concentric or eccentric. In concentric dynamic contractions, the muscle length shortens on generating force. In eccentric dynamic contractions, the muscle lengthens in response to a greater opposing force.[12]

Another form of RET is high-velocity resistance training also known as power training. It involves the use of high-speed contractions at low external resistances (40% of one-repetition maximum [1RM]), commonly in the concentric component. Some studies in older adults suggest that this form of RET may be more relevant because the progressive decline in muscle power is more rapid and occurs sooner than the decline in muscle strength, making muscle power a more critical variable for functionality.[16,17]

What is the Evidence?

The effects of RET can be assessed by evaluating muscle strength and power, which are characteristics associated with functional performance. There are several methods available, including isometric, isotonic, isokinetic, 1-RM, multiple RM (3-RM), stair climbing, and vertical jump protocols. There is high-quality evidence that RET programs, although to a variable extent, produce substantial increases in muscle strength and power in older adults.[9,15] Variations in these changes depend on factors such as sex, type and duration of intervention, and specific muscle groups examined. The benefits of RET on other characteristics, such as body composition, muscle quality, and muscle endurance, have also been studied. Some reports show favorable changes of moderate-high intensity RET in body composition measured by an increase in fat-free mass and a decrease in total body fat.[9,14] Improvements in muscle quality after RET, when evaluating increased motor unit recruitment and discharge rates, have shown similar benefits in older adults to those seen in younger adults. Muscular endurance has also shown improvement after moderate-high–intensity RET.[9]

Benefits in Chronic Disease

Strengthening exercise programs for the core and hip muscles can improve the mobility of older adults, reduce kyphotic posturing, and reduce the risk of osteoporotic vertebral fractures.[18] High-intensity RET has been demonstrated to improve bone mineral density in lumbar and femoral bones.[9] RET is preferred over endurance exercises for maintaining bone mass, and progressive resistance exercises may also induce osteogenesis. In older adults, weakness and poor recruitment of the paraspinal muscles will diminish their protective role on the spine. This diminishment can be related to further kyphotic or scoliotic deformities and augment the risk for vertebral fractures. RET with focus on strengthening the back extensors can be beneficial in the management of osteoporosis, especially in postmenopausal women. The benefits of these exercises in the prevention of osteoporotic fractures may be independent of the effects on bone mineral density and can also be related to a decrease in the risk of falling.[18]

In older patients with osteoarthritis, strengthening exercises also have favorable benefits. There is high-quality evidence supporting the use of RET programs for persons with hip and knee osteoarthritis to reduce symptoms of pain and improving physical function and general QOL.[19,20] Aquatic exercises provide natural resistance from water and also take a load off from the joints and bones. There is moderate-quality evidence of the benefits of aquatic exercises for hip and knee osteoarthritis.[21]

Exercise Recommendations

The initial strengthening exercise program in older adults should start with low intensity (40%–50% of 1RM, or exercising to the point of fatigue). If the person is in pain or has considerable weakness when performing the exercise, isometric strengthening should be used. If the person has more exercise experience or when the pain and weakness improve, the program should progress to moderate (60%–70% of 1RM) and high-intensity (80% of 1RM) exercises that have shown more health benefits as previously mentioned. These exercises should be performed 2 to 3 times per week, 10 to 15 repetitions; the major muscle groups should be addressed, including the core and hip muscles, which are essential for prevention of falls.[3,9,12,18] Complementing traditional RET with high-velocity power training should be considered for a more optimal training method.[16,22] Aquatic resistance exercises should be considered as an alternative for older adults with poor balance and conditions that may limit weight-bearing activity.

FLEXIBILITY/STRETCHING
Basic Concepts

Flexibility is the range of motion (ROM) in a joint or in a group of joints. It is influenced by muscles, tendons, and bones and is described as the degree to which muscle length permits movement over the joint in which it has influence.[12] It has been postulated that by 70 years of age, flexibility and joint ROM declines are significant for hip (20%–30%), spine (20%–30%), and ankle (30%–40%), especially in women.[9] To help reduce such decrease in flexibility and ROM, stretching has been seen to provide elongation of soft tissues and an increase in muscle length.[12]

There are several types of flexibility exercises described in literature that can improve ROM:

1. Dynamic stretching involves a gradual transition from one body position to another and a progressive increase in reach and ROM as the movement is repeated several times.
2. Static stretching involves slowly stretching a muscle/tendon group and holding the position for a period of time. It can be divided into
   a. Active: involves holding the stretched position using the strength of the agonist muscle
   b. Passive: involves holding the limb or other part of the body with or without the assistance of a partner or device
3. Proprioceptive neuromuscular facilitation methods typically involve an isometric contraction of the selected muscle-tendon group followed by a static stretching of the same group.
4. Ballistic methods use the momentum of the moving body segment to produce the stretch in a bouncing motion.
   a. This method is generally not recommended for everyday people who want to stay in shape or improve flexibility because there is a risk of straining or pulling a muscle because of the high speed of the movements. If done, they should be performed only under the supervision of a professional.

Flexibility measurements include flexion and extension movements, but there are no current tests available that can provide representative values of total body flexibility. Because flexibility is joint specific, determining the ROM in a joint does not necessarily indicate the level of flexibility in other joints. Currently, the most reliable and accurate measures to confirm flexibility are those whereby a goniometer is used to measure the actual degrees of rotation of various joints.

What is the Evidence?

There are only a few studies that have been able to describe or compare the effects of specific ROM exercises on flexibility outcomes in older populations. Chodzko-Zajko and colleagues[9] describe a study whereby significant improvements are seen in low-back/hamstring flexibility and spinal extension after 10 weeks of a supervised static stretching program that involved a series of low-back and hip exercises in 70-year-old women. Although there is not enough evidence that demonstrates the beneficial effects of stretching in injury prevention, it has been recognized that chronic stretching effectually can improve joint ROM.[23]

Studies have shown that the decreased flexibility in the elderly also decreases their ability to recover quickly from a perturbation. Lack of necessary ROM would decrease the effectiveness of hip and ankle strategies. If a person is unable to counteract a perturbation due to lack of flexibility and lack of appropriate ROM, the perturbation may result in a fall. Such findings have been described in prior studies whereby a correlation has been found between short hip and ankle muscles and increased falls in the elderly.[23]

Benefits in Chronic Disease

Poor joint flexibility in addition to muscle tightness, especially in the hamstring groups, can be a predisposing factor in increased risk of joint and muscle injuries.[24] Researchers have shown that 12 months of stretching is as effective as strengthening exercises or manual therapy in patients with chronic neck pain. Lewit and colleagues and Simons and colleagues[25] reported an immediate 94% reduction in pain associated with trigger points after applying a special technique based on the stretching principle. For this, stretching is now being incorporated as a crucial component in pain management programs.

Exercise Recommendations

Flexibility exercise refers to activities designed to preserve or extend ROM around a joint.[9] Holding a stretch for 10 to 30 seconds at the point of tightness or slight discomfort enhances joint ROM, with little apparent benefit resulting from longer durations. Older persons may realize greater improvements in ROM with longer durations (30–60 seconds) of stretching. Repeating each flexibility exercise 2 to 4 times is effective, with enhancement of joint ROM occurring at 3 to 12 weeks, if done at a frequency of at least 2 to 3 times a week; greater gain is reached if done on a daily basis. The goal is to attain 60 seconds of total stretching time per flexibility exercise, resting between stretches for about 30 to 60 seconds. One must adjust duration and repetitions according to individual needs.[26] In older patients, activities that maintain or increase flexibility using sustained stretches of moderate intensity for each major muscle group and static rather than ballistic movements is preferred.[9,26] Further research is needed before making universal recommendations concerning the timing of stretching in association with other exercise activities. Nonetheless, based on the available evidence, those engaging in a general fitness program should perform flexibility exercises after cardiorespiratory or resistance exercise or as a stand-alone program.[26]

STABILITY/BALANCE
Basic Concepts

Balance is the ability to maintain the body's center of mass (COM) within the limits of the base of support. Balance disorders in the geriatric population are often a multifactorial condition. Weakness in the core stabilizing muscles, altered muscle activation patterns, loss of proprioception, and an inability to control normal postural control can all result in decreased balance in the elderly.[27] Joint stability is achieved by the combination of static and dynamic components. Static stability is obtained through the structural stability offered by structures such as bones, capsules, and ligaments. Dynamic stability refers to the neuromuscular control of the skeletal muscle affecting a joint to maintain its center of rotation in response to perturbation.[12] There are 3 different strategies described to maintain a straight posture: ankle, hip, and step strategies. Hip and ankle strategies include activation of the muscles opposite to the direction of the perturbation. The step strategy is initiated once the magnitude of the perturbation is too big. It starts by taking a step in the direction of the perturbation, which allows preservation of the COM and, thus, an undisturbed balance.[23]

Various measures have been described to determine patients' balance and stability. The Sensory Organization Test measures the ability to use somatosensory, visual, and vestibular information to control the body while standing. The Limits of Stability test is a dynamic test that measures the ability to shift the body's weight in different directions while maintaining stability.[28] The Berg Balance Scale is a 14-item objective measure designed to assess static balance and fall risk in adult populations. The Functional Gait Assessment helps assess postural stability during various walking tasks. Patients' locomotor function can be measured using such tests as the 6-minute walk and timed get up and go.

What is the Evidence?

The evidence for the benefits of specific balance training exercises is scarce. There is modest evidence that balance exercises included in a multimodal exercise program with strengthening exercises have shown to decrease fall risk.[9] Tsang and Hui-Chan[28] found that subjects who performed 4 weeks of intensive tai chi demonstrated an improvement in sensory organization test, especially the vestibular component, and in the limits of stability test measures. Also, the improved balance control exhibited by tai chi participants led to a decrease in multiple fall risk by 47.5%. More data are still needed in order to better understand the benefits and effectiveness of balance training programs in the elderly population.

Benefits in Chronic Disease

Balance strategy training (BST) exercises can be beneficial for improving balance, strength, and overall functional ability in various populations, such as the elderly, osteopenic adults, and menopausal women. Also, BST may be a promising intervention strategy to improve balance and strength in patients with myasthenia gravis by improving balance and quantitative myasthenia gravis scores.[29] Li and colleagues[30] showed that in patients with mild to moderate Parkinson disease, participating in tai chi training led to reduced balance impairments, reduced falls, and improvements in functional capacity.

Exercise Recommendations

Exercise prescription guidelines recommend using activities that include the following: progressively difficult postures that gradually reduce the base of support (2-legged stand to 1-legged stand), dynamic movements that perturb the center of gravity (circle turns), stressing postural muscle groups (toe stands), or reducing sensory input (standing with eyes closed). Balance training activities, such as lower-body strengthening and walking over difficult terrain, have been shown to significantly improve balance in many studies.[9] Stability and balance programs in healthy adults should be performed 2 to 3 days per week, particularly for older adults who want to improve function and prevent falls. Initially, single muscles are isolated with the goal of combining several muscles in simple movements in stable positions and in a single cardinal plane. The program's difficulty is increased by increasing speed, adding multidirectional movements, adding off-axis loads in all cardinal planes, and adding progressively unstable surfaces. Progression to a higher level of stability should only be done when patients have adequately completed the previous level, being careful not to add external instability onto internal instability.[12] Neuromotor exercise training, such as tai chi, qigong, and yoga, incorporate motor skills, such as balance, coordination, gait, agility, and proprioceptive training, which help improve balance, agility, muscle strength, and reduce the risk of falls.[27]

Occupational therapy (OT) treatments for balance disorders and fall prevention include increasing postural stability and strength, upper-extremity strength and endurance, proprioceptive awareness, and safe functional mobility. Functional standing tasks, such as emptying the dishwasher, can promote dynamic standing strength and proprioceptive awareness, increasing strength and endurance in postural muscles. OT can also educate patients on energy conservation and safety techniques. Activities that require dynamic standing balance, such as lower-body dressing and bathing tasks, are also functional ways to increase balance and safety as well as independence (**Table 1**).[27]

Table 1 Recommendations for exercise activity in older adults	
Type of Exercise	**Aerobic**
Program	Continuous exercise (eg, running, fast walking, cycling, rowing, swimming)
Frequency	3–5 d/wk
Intensity	Moderate (50%–60% Vo_{2max})
	High (70%–80% Vo_{2max})
Repetitions	30 min (moderate) or 20 min (vigorous). Can also do 10 min bouts x 3
Type of Exercise	**Resistance**
Program	Free weights
	Resistance bands
	Progressive resistance exercises combined with power training
Frequency	2–3 d/wk
Intensity	Start low (40% 1RM) progress to moderate (60% 1RM) and high (80% 1RM)
	Power training (20%–40% 1RM)
Repetitions	2–3 sets of 8–12 repetitions addressing major muscle groups, including core and hips.
Type of Exercise	**Flexibility**
Program	Static stretching preferred over ballistic stretching
Frequency	$\geq$2–3 d/wk
Intensity	Stretch to point of tightness or mild discomfort
Repetitions	2–4 of each stretch; resting between stretches for 30–60 s
Type of Exercise	**Balance**
Program	Proprioceptive training, agility, gait, tai chi, yoga, progressive difficult postures, perturbation exercises, sensory input reduction (eyes closed)
Frequency	$\geq$2–3 d/wk

Adapted from Chodzko-Zajko WJ, Proctor DN, Fiatarone Singh MA, et al. Exercise and physical activity for older adults. Med Sci Sports Exerc 2009;41(7):1510–30; and Garber CE, Blissmer B, Deschenes MR, et al. Quantity and quality of exercise for developing and maintaining cardiorespiratory, musculoskeletal, and neuromotor fitness in apparently healthy adults: guidance for prescribing exercise. Med Sci Sports Exerc 2011;43(7):1334–59, with permission.

BENEFITS OF EXERCISE ON COGNITION AND QUALITY OF LIFE

A physically active lifestyle promotes feelings of well-being and improved QOL and is associated with a lower risk of cognitive decline and dementia.[26] The mechanism for the relationship between physical activity, exercise, and cognitive functioning is not well understood; but it has been suggested that enhanced blood flow, increased brain volume, elevations in brain-derived neurotropic factor, and improvements in neurotransmitter systems and IGF-1 function may occur in response to behavioral and aerobic training.[9] On the other hand, improvements in mood are proposed to be caused by exercise-induced increase in blood circulation to the brain and by the hypothalamic-pituitary-adrenal axis influence with other regions of the brain that control mood (limbic system), stress (amygdala), and motivation (hippocampus).[31]

An acute exposure to a single bout of aerobic exercise can result in short-term improvements in memory, attention, and reaction time; aerobic exercise plus resistive exercise training can produce improvements in anxiety, depression, overall well-being, and QOL.[9] Scully and colleagues[32] describe that those with depression respond well to aerobic exercises conducted at 60% to 70% of maximal heart rate, 2 to 5 times a week for 30 to 40 minutes, with most anxiolytic effects seen with short bouts in programs performed for several months (>9 weeks).

Overall it can be seen that a physically active lifestyle, either through aerobic or resistive exercise, can help in treating and even preventing relapses of multiple cognitive and physiologic conditions when performed at a certain intensity, frequency, and duration.

BENEFITS OF SPORTS PARTICIPATION

Organized sports participation plays an important role in promoting exercise activity in older adults. Common sports like swimming, cycling, running, aerobics, soccer, and racquet sports have proven beneficial for improving all-cause mortality and cardiovascular risks.[33] In addition to the benefits on physical function and general QOL, playing team sports contributes more to the person's motivation compared with individual exercise activity in older adults.[34] This benefit may be associated with the social interactions during team sports activity.

PRECAUTIONS AND BARRIERS

Older adults who are planning to participate in an exercise program should undergo preparticipation screening to evaluate potential risks (mostly cardiovascular) that may require specific modifications to the exercise prescription. Uncontrolled hypertension, unstable angina, third-degree heart block, recent myocardial infarction, or acute heart failure are absolute contraindications to exercise in older adults.[2] Other factors, such as balance problems, visual deficits, polypharmacy use, and peripheral vascular and neuropathic disease, should also be assessed. Education regarding proper hydration and nutrition during exercise should be provided because the thirst mechanism in older adults is less sensitive.[3] Exercise may increase the risk of musculoskeletal injury. Performing warm-ups and cooldowns, flexibility, and gradual progression of volume and intensity should help reduce these risks.[26] Musculoskeletal pain or disability has been cited as a reason for not exercising in up to half of older adults, whereas habit is the single best predictor of inactivity.[2] Overcoming habitual inactivity is one of the most important challenges we face when prescribing an exercise program to older adults.

SUMMARY

There is outstanding evidence that exercise activity has many favorable benefits for older adults, improving physical function, cardiovascular risk factors, all-cause mortality, and general QOL, among others. The exercise recommendations should be individually tailored to the abilities, precautions, and goals of each person. The ideal program should include components of aerobic, resistance, flexibility, and balance training exercises. They also should be of sufficient intensity, volume, and duration in order to achieve maximal benefits. As physiatrists, we should be leaders promoting exercise activity to our older population, not only for therapeutic purposes but also as prevention and risk reduction of their coming changes with aging.

REFERENCES

1. U.S. Census Bureau. The older population: 2010. 2010 census briefs. 2011. 1–19. Available at: https://www.census.gov/newsroom/releases/archives/2010_census/cb11-cn192.html.
2. Nied R, Franklin B. Promoting and prescribing exercise for the elderly. Am Fam Physician 2002;65(3):419–26.

3. Concannon LG, Grierson MJ, Harrast MA. Exercise in the older adult: from the sedentary elderly to the masters athlete [Theme issue: exercise and sports]. PM R 2012;4(11):833–9. Elsevier Inc.

4. Wullems JA, Verschueren SMP, Degens H, et al. A review of the assessment and prevalence of sedentarism in older adults, its physiology/health impact and non-exercise mobility counter-measures. Biogerontology 2016;17:547–65.

5. Nelson ME, Rejeski WJ, Blair SN, et al. Physical activity and public health in older adults: recommendation from the American College of Sports Medicine and the American Heart Association. Med Sci Sports Exerc 2007;39(8):1435–45.

6. Seals DR, Walker AE, Pierce GL, et al. Habitual exercise and vascular ageing. J Physiol 2009;587(Pt 23):5541–9.

7. Evans WJ. Protein nutrition, exercise and aging. J Am Coll Nutr 2004;23(6 Suppl): 601S–9S. Available at: http://www.ncbi.nlm.nih.gov/pubmed/15640513. Accessed February 28, 2017.

8. Rivera-Brown AM, Frontera WR. Principles of exercise physiology: responses to acute exercise and long-term adaptations to training. PM R 2012;4(11): 797–804. Elsevier Inc.

9. Chodzko-Zajko WJ, Proctor DN, Fiatarone Singh MA, et al. Exercise and physical activity for older adults. Med Sci Sports Exerc 2009;41(7):1510–30.

10. Villareal DT, Chode S, Parimi N, et al. Weight loss, exercise, or both and physical function in obese older adults. N Engl J Med 2011;364(13):1218–29. Available at: http://www.ncbi.nlm.nih.gov/pubmed/21449785%5Cnhttp://www.pubmedcentral. nih.gov/articlerender.fcgi?artid=PMC3114602.

11. Santos-Parker JR, LaRocca TJ, Seals DR. Aerobic exercise and other healthy life-style factors that influence vascular aging. Adv Physiol Educ 2014;38(4): 296–307. Available at: http://www.ncbi.nlm.nih.gov/pubmed/25434012.

12. Micheo W, Baerga L, Miranda G. Basic principles regarding strength, flexibility, and stability exercises. PM R 2012;4(11):805–11. Elsevier Inc.

13. Snijders T, Verdijk LB, van Loon LJC. The impact of sarcopenia and exercise training on skeletal muscle satellite cells. Ageing Res Rev 2009;8:328–38.

14. Stewart VH, Saunders DH, Greig CA. Responsiveness of muscle size and strength to physical training in very elderly people: a systematic review. Scand J Med Sci Sports 2014;24(1):1–10.

15. Churchward-venne TA, Tieland M, Verdijk LB, et al. There are no nonresponders to resistance-type exercise training in older men and women. J Am Med Dir Assoc 2015;16(5):400–11. Elsevier Inc.

16. Sayers SP, Gibson K. A comparison of high-speed power training and tradi-tional slow-speed resistance training in older men and women. J Strength Cond Res 2010;24(12):3369–80. Available at: http://www.ncbi.nlm.nih.gov/ pubmed/21068681.

17. Buford TW, Anton SD, Clark DJ, et al. Optimizing the benefits of exercise on phys-ical function in older adults. PM R 2014;6:528–43.

18. Sinaki M. Exercise for patients with osteoporosis: management of vertebral compression fractures and trunk strengthening for fall prevention. PM R 2012; 4(11):882–8. Elsevier Inc.

19. Fransen M, McConnell S, Hernandez-Molina G, et al. Exercise for osteoarthritis of the hip. Cochrane Database Syst Rev 2014;(4). CD007912. Available at: http://www.ncbi.nlm.nih.gov/entrez/query.fcgi?cmd=Retrieve&db=PubMed&dopt= Citation&list_uids=12918008.

20. Fransen M, McConnell S, Harmer A. Exercise for osteoarthritis of the knee. Cochrane Database Syst Rev 2015;(1). CD004376. Available at: http://www.ncbi.nlm.nih.gov/pubmed/27015856.
21. Bartels E, Juhl C, Christensen R. Aquatic exercise for osteoarthritis of the knee or hip. Cochrane Database Syst Rev 2016;(3). CD005523. Available at: http://bjsm.bmj.com/.
22. Sayers S. High-speed power training: a novel approach to resistance training in older men and women. A brief review and pilot study. J Strength Cond Res 2007; 21(2):518–26.
23. Reddy RS, Alahmari KA. Effect of lower extremity stretching exercises on balance in geriatric population. Int J Health Sci (Qassim) 2016;10(3):389–95. Available at: http://www.ncbi.nlm.nih.gov/pubmed/27610062%5Cnhttp://www.pubmedcentral.nih.gov/articlerender.fcgi?artid=PMC5003582.
24. Onigbinde AT, Akindoyi O, Faremi FA, et al. An assessment of hamstring flexibility of subjects with knee osteoarthritis and their age matched control. Clin Med Res 2013;2(6):121–5.
25. Page P. Current concepts in muscle stretching for exercise and rehabilitation. Int J Sports Phys Ther 2016;7(1):109.
26. Garber CE, Blissmer B, Deschenes MR, et al. Quantity and quality of exercise for developing and maintaining cardiorespiratory, musculoskeletal, and neuromotor fitness in apparently healthy adults: guidance for prescribing exercise. Med Sci Sports Exerc 2011;43(7):1334–59.
27. Enix DE, Schulz J, Flaherty JH, et al. Balance problems in the geriatric patient. Top Integr Heal Care Int J 2011;2(1):1–10. Available at: http://www.tihcij.com/Articles/Balance-Problems-in-the-Geriatric-Patient.aspx?id=0000256.
28. Tsang WWN, Hui-Chan CWY. Effect of 4- and 8-wk intensive tai chi training on balance control in the elderly. Med Sci Sports Exerc 2004;36(4):648–57.
29. Wong SH, Nitz JC, Williams K, et al. Effects of balance strategy training in myasthenia gravis: a case study series. Muscle Nerve 2014;49(5):654–60.
30. Li F, Harmer P, FitzGerald K, et al. Tai chi and postural stability in patients with Parkinson's disease. N Engl J Med 2012;366(6):511–9. Available at: http://www.nejm.org/doi/full/10.1056/NEJMoa1107911.
31. Sharma A, Madaan V, Petty FD. Exercise for mental health. Prim Care Companion J Clin Psychiatry 2006;8(2):106. Available at: http://www.pubmedcentral.nih.gov/articlerender.fcgi?artid=1470658&tool=pmcentrez&rendertype=abstract.
32. Scully D, Kremer J, Meade MM, et al. Physical exercise and psychological well being: a critical review. Br J Sports Med 1998;32(2):111–20.
33. Oja P, Kelly P, Pedisic Z, et al. Associations of specific types of sports and exercise with all-cause and cardiovascular-disease mortality: a cohort study of 80 306 British adults. Br J Sports Med 2017;51(10):812–7. Available at: http://www.ncbi.nlm.nih.gov/pubmed/27895075.
34. Pedersen MT, Vorup J, Nistrup A, et al. Effect of team sports and resistance training on physical function, quality of life, and motivation in older adults. Scand J Med Sci Sports 2017;27(8):852–64. Available at: http://doi.wiley.com/10.1111/sms.12823.

Alternative Treatment Modalities and Its Effect in Older Populations

Carlos E. Rivera-Tavarez, MD

KEYWORDS

- Health span • Aging • Antiaging • Alternative exercises • Longevity

KEY POINTS

- Preventive measures are an indispensable part of promoting a healthier aging process.
- Careful attention to nutrition, environmental factors, and lifestyle could lead to a longer health span.
- As we age, more leisure time is available and the risk of a sedentary life increases; exercise is a very powerful promoter of health.
- Diet modifications and the use of supplements show promise in decreasing chronic inflammation by activating antioxidant pathways.
- Activity, alternative exercises, meditation, and sleep can all affect and improve our health span.

ALTERNATIVE TREATMENT MODALITIES AND THEIR EFFECT IN OLDER POPULATIONS

According to the Centers for Disease Control and Prevention, most of the leading causes of death are result of chronic conditions. Aging leads to lower physical activity (PA) and PA options.[1] In adults aged 65 years and older, PA includes leisure time PA (for example, walking, dancing, gardening, hiking, swimming), transportation (eg, walking or cycling), occupational (if the individual is still engaged in work), household chores, play, games, sports or planned exercise, in the context of daily, family, and community activities (World Health Organization).[2] In order to improve cardiorespiratory and muscular fitness and bone and functional health and reduce the risk of noncommunicable diseases, depression, and cognitive decline, the American College of Sports Medicine recommends[3] the following:

- Older adults should do at least 150 minutes of moderate-intensity aerobic PA throughout the week or do at least 75 minutes of vigorous-intensity aerobic PA

Disclosure statement: The author has nothing to disclose.
Campbell Clinic Orthopedics, 8000 Centerview Parkway, Suite 500, Memphis, TN 38018, USA
E-mail address: crivera@campbellclinic.com

Phys Med Rehabil Clin N Am 28 (2017) 671–680
http://dx.doi.org/10.1016/j.pmr.2017.06.002
1047-9651/17/© 2017 Elsevier Inc. All rights reserved.

throughout the week or an equivalent combination of moderate- and vigorous-intensity activity.
- Aerobic activity should be performed in bouts of at least 10 minutes' duration.
- For additional health benefits, older adults should increase their moderate-intensity aerobic PA to 300 minutes per week or engage in 150 minutes of vigorous-intensity aerobic PA per week or an equivalent combination of moderate- and vigorous-intensity activity.
- Older adults, with poor mobility, should perform PA to enhance balance and prevent falls on 3 or more days per week.
- Neuromotor exercise (sometimes called functional fitness training) is recommended for 20 to 30 minutes per day, 2 or 3 days per week. Exercises should involve motor skills (balance, agility, coordination, and gait), proprioceptive exercise training, and multifaceted activities (tai chi and yoga) to improve physical function and prevent falls in older adults.

When older adults cannot do the recommended amounts of PA because of health conditions, they should be as physically active as their abilities and conditions allow. There is a consistency of findings across studies and a range of outcome measures related to functional independence; regular aerobic activity and short-term exercise programs confer a reduced risk of functional limitations and disability in older age. Although a precise characterization of a minimal or effective PA dose to maintain functional independence is difficult, it seems moderate to higher levels of activity are effective and there may be a threshold of at least moderate activity for significant outcomes.[4] PA improves overall life satisfaction and enjoyment. As we age we also face barriers to staying physically active. These barriers include economic constraints, lack of social resources, retirement, living on a fix income, health, and death of spouse, among others. Moderate to vigorous PA and cardiorespiratory fitness have been independently, statistically significantly associated with reduce risk of mortality.[5] Whereas high individual variations are inherent to the response to exercise, most studies have reported that exercise can attenuate motor and cognitive declines associated with aging and dementia.[6]

Even though aerobic and resistance exercises are the best known and more commonly practiced forms of exercise, other alternatives with lower-impact activities and exercises have shown great success in older adults. Cognitive aging is the cognitive decline seen in aging in the absence of specific dementia characteristics. It is not certain what we can do to maintain mental abilities; but certain exercise programs and practices may be helpful, as most types of supplements have failed to show any consistent benefits.

Tai Chi

- It is a multicomponent mind and body exercise that is grounded in the holistic model of traditional Chinese medicine. Tai chi (TC) is a form of meditation in motion, the idea of challenging the body to stay centered and balanced while moving and concentrating on several things at once.
- The gentle nature of TC makes it a natural physical therapy tool for people with joint problems, low bone density, Parkinson disease (PD), and other ailments. Connection to the breath is vital to healing, enhanced balance, and flexibility. Many TC stances increase leg strength and develop the muscles to protect fragile joints, such as the knees and hips. This activity is very beneficial for mature adults and seniors. It is a safe activity with high levels of adherence and enjoyment.

- TC is reported to improve symptoms and systems associated with age-related decline, including cardiovascular (CV) function, balance, gait, cognitive functioning, self-efficacy, and quality of life (QOL).[7]
- TC is based on slow intentional movements, often coordinated with breathing and imagery, that aims to strengthen and relax the physical body and mind, enhance the natural flow of life (qi), and improve health, personal development, and, in some systems, self-defense.[7]
- It has been shown to lead to improvements in indicators of cognitive function and maintain improvements through 12 months.[8]
- Falls are common among older adults and are one of the major threats to their health. The incidence of falls varies with living status and increases with age; in the general population, 30% to 40% of people older than 65 years fall every year worldwide, increasing to approximately 50% among people aged 80 years and older. Falls in older people are associated with considerable subsequent decline in functional status and increase in nursing home admissions and medical resource consumption. Fall-related complications are the leading cause of unintentional injury deaths in people older than 65 years and the fifth leading cause of death. A recent systemic review and meta-analysis showed that TC exercise is effective for preventing falls in older adults. This preventive effect seems to increase with exercise frequency.[9]
- Another important benefit is improvement in sleep quality. This improvement has been shown in older adults even with cognitive impairment. Their sleep duration, efficiency, and the mental health component of QOL can also improve with this type of exercise.[10] Important aspects about sleep and circadian rhythm are discussed later.
- In patients with CV disease (CVD), TC could provide more benefits than other exercises or no intervention for decreasing both systolic and diastolic blood pressure and improving biochemical outcomes, physical function, QOL, and depression.[11]

Yoga

- Yoga is an ancient Indian way of life that includes changes in mental attitude and the practice of specific techniques, such as postures, breathing patterns, and meditation, to attain the highest levels of consciousness.[12]
- Yoga is a psychosomatic spiritual discipline for achieving union and harmony between our mind, body, and soul and the ultimate union of our individual consciousness with the universal consciousness.
- When a person practices yoga with yogic attitude (patience, persistence, overcoming obstacles within self), there are several changes in physiology.[12]
  - It improves the sensibility of B cells in the pancreas to glucose signals and improves insulin sensitivity.
  - Deep breathing patterns stretch lung tissues; this can synchronize neural elements with concomitant changes in the autonomic nervous system, reducing metabolism and stimulating the parasympathetic system.
  - It can interact with autonomic centers and increase melatonin levels.[13]
  - Meditators have shown larger gray matter volumes and brain changes in areas involved with sensory, cognitive, and emotional processing.
  - Meditators experience better QOL and functional health.
  - During meditation heart rate, oxygen consumption and respiratory rate decrease in experienced practitioners.

- Meditators have also shown better scores in attention, concentration tasks, as well as fine coordinated movements; studies have shown positive effects in patients with respiratory disease and CVDs as well as diabetic patients and people with joint disorders.
- It can decrease indices of oxidative stress.[14]
  - It can reduce the metabolic rate by as much as 40% to 64%, which is within ranges of hibernating animals.
  - A single 20-minute session of yogic breathing practice could reduce the levels of key proinflammatory biomarkers in saliva.[15]

Meditation

- Active-based meditations can have effects in many areas of the brain; meditative practices commonly affect brain systems involved in attention, memory, conscious awareness, reward, and emotional regulation that are important and can be disrupted by cerebrovascular and neurodegenerative changes.[16]
- Clinical research now suggests that meditation-based practices may be an effective means of addressing anxiety,[17] depression, and substance abuse.[18]
- Meditation reduced all subjects' pain intensity and unpleasantness ratings with decreases ranging from 11% to 70% and from 20% to 93%, respectively. Moreover, meditation-related pain relief was directly related to brain regions associated with the cognitive modulation of pain.[19]
- Even though it is very difficult to compare meditation studies because of different techniques and methods, there have been studies on the influence of meditation on cognitive functions in the context of aging and neurodegenerative diseases; the results imply a positive effect, especially on attention, memory, verbal fluency, and cognitive flexibility.[20]
  - The mechanisms include increased cerebral perfusion in prefrontal, parietal, and auditory cortex; a protective effect on gray matter thickness; and enhancing of the function of areas involved in attention. In addition, meditation can potentially enhance the power of cognitive circuits and increase cognitive capacity. Moreover, it can improve myelination or restructuralization of white-matter tracts in the involved areas, such as the anterior corona radiata associated with the anterior cingulate cortex.[16]
  - Another explanation of the neuroprotective effect of meditation can be the decrease in cortisol level caused by stress. Meditation can positively impact dyslipidemia and oxidative stress, which further decreases the risk of vascular diseases of the brain as well as Alzheimer disease.
  - From a psychological point of view, the effects on cognitive functions can be explained by enhancing the ability of mindfulness. Mindfulness enables a nonjudgmental reflection of processes happening in consciousness beyond concrete contents of thoughts and feelings. This reflection leads to experiencing a relativity and transient nature of these contents, which can form the long-term point of view, lead to weakening of affective power of these perceptions in consciousness (eg, as in anxiety), and enlarge the capacity for focused processing. This ability can lead to improvement in attentional and working memory tasks.
- Meditative practices may be especially useful in aging adults for several reasons. It involves low-impact activities that can be tolerated by everyone, even older adults with physical limitations, without adverse events. It can be adapted to sitting and lying down positions if necessary. It improves mood and ability to cope with chronic stress, provides relief of chronic pain, and can reduce polypharmacy.[20]

Dance

- Dance is a very affordable, accessible, and socially engaging mode of physical activity. It challenges dynamic balance and stimulates strength, flexibility, and endurance.
- Among multiple leisure time PAs (tennis, golf, dancing, walking), only dance reduced the risk of dementia.[21]
  - This finding could be due to increase neuroplasticity stimulated by the complex interaction of movement and thought processes during dancing. A dance style that promotes split-second decision-making is better than a style based on memorized paths.
- In patients with PD, dance interventions have shown to improve many motor functions like upper extremity control, proprioception, and some gait parameters.[22] Also positive effects on social life, everyday life competence, functional mobility (rigidity, fine motor skills, and facial expression), and QOL of patients and their caregivers have been demonstrated.[23]
- A combination of dance and relaxation exercises improves QOL and cognitive impairment and reduces anxiety and depression among cognitively impaired elderly residents of government institutions as compared with relaxation alone.[24]
- Dance also showed improvement in episodic memory over a general health education program.[25]

Music

- Postexercise parasympathetic reactivation seems to be an important mechanism with a cardioprotective effect in both healthy and cardiovascularly compromised people. Physical exercise increases sympathetic and decreased parasympathetic stimuli, resulting in increased heart rate that rapidly declines after cessation of exercise by parasympathetic reactivation. Blunted reactivation of the parasympathetic system has been reported in patients with congestive heart failure and coronary artery disease, and this increases the risk of sudden death.
- Music has been shown to be an effective, safe, low-cost method of modulating emotions and autonomic nervous system (ANS) activity. In healthy adults, it shifts the autonomic balance to parasympathetic predominance. After listening to music, the parasympathetic nervous system activity is increased. This increase produces an attenuation of the exercise-induce decrease in heart rate variability.[26]
- Combining physical exercises with music produces more positive effects on cognitive function in elderly people than exercise alone. This effect can be attributed to the multifaceted nature of combining physical exercise with music, which can act simultaneously as both cognitive and physical training.[27]
- Levitin and Chanda[28] found that music improves the body's immune system function and reduces stress. Listening to music was also found to be more effective than prescription drugs in reducing anxiety before surgery. Music also reduces levels of the stress hormone cortisol.

Heat Exposure/Sauna

- Heat stress will activate genes that make heat shock proteins (HSPs). HSPs are molecular chaperones that protect the proteome by folding denatured polypeptides and promoting the degradation of severely damaged proteins.[29] HSPs decrease protein aggregation that is seen in heart and neurodegenerative diseases. A genotype associated with HSP is more likely in centenarians. The heat shock response declines in potency over the lifetime; enfeeblement of the response contributes to aging by permitting the emergence of protein aggregation diseases, reduction in cellular vigor, and decreased longevity.[29]

- In rats, daily heat stress treatment (40°C, 30 m/d) rescues denervation-induced loss of mitochondria and concomitant muscle atrophy. It was also found that denervation-activated autophagy-dependent mitochondrial clearance (mitophagy) was suppressed by daily heat stress treatment. The molecular basis of this observation is explained by showing that heat stress treatment attenuates the increase of key proteins that regulate the tagging step for mitochondrial clearance and the intermediate step of autophagosome formation in denervated muscle. These findings contribute to the better understanding of mitochondrial quality control in denervated muscle from a translational perspective and provide a mechanism behind the attenuation of muscle wasting by heat stress.[30]
- Passive environmental heat stress (up to 30 minutes at 73°C) increases motor cortical excitability and enhances performance in a motor skill acquisition task.[31]
- During sauna sessions, heart rate may increase to more than 100 to 150 beats per minute, which corresponds to a moderate-vigorous physical activity. Also 30- to 60-minute sessions can increase growth hormone levels 2 to 4 fold. Sauna use (80°C–100°C, at least 20 minutes) decreases total mortality by 24% if used 2 to 3 times per week and 40% if used 4 to 7 times per week. Increased frequency of sauna bathing is associated with a reduced risk of sudden cardiac death, CVD, and all-cause mortality.[29]

Cryotherapy

- Whole-body cryotherapy treatments consist of applying short cryogenic temperatures (less than −100°C) to the whole body of patients in order to induce a physiologic response. Cryotherapy results in a reduction in the frequency and degree of pain perception in patients with osteoarthritis. A 10-day cycle of cold treatment reduced the number of analgesic medications in these patients. Cryotherapy treatments improved the range of PA and had a positive effect on the well-being of the patients.[32]
- A single whole-body cryotherapy (3 minutes at −110°C in a cryochamber) or partial body cryotherapy (3 minutes at −160°C in an open tank) session induces an immediate stimulation of the ANS with a predominance of the parasympathetic tone.[33]
  - Elevated parasympathetic activity at rest is classically associated with health and well-being and is stimulated by regular physical activity. In the immediate postexercise period, an increase in the parasympathetic modulation of the heart rate is also a crucial physiologic reaction necessary to initiate cardio-deceleration and a complete recovery. Conversely, a delayed or incomplete parasympathetic reactivation after exercise is associated with impaired recovery as well as with an increased risk of ventricular fibrillation and sudden cardiac death. Thus, parasympathetic activity is thought to afford a cardioprotective background and is probably a valid indicator of postexercise recovery in athletes.
- There is an inverse relationship between brown adipose tissue (BAT) activity and body fatness suggesting that BAT, because of its energy-dissipating activity, is protective against body fat accumulation. Cold exposure activates and recruits BAT in association with increased energy expenditure and decreased body fatness. The stimulatory effects of cold are mediated through transient receptor potential (TRP) channels, most of which are also chemesthetic receptors for various food ingredients. In fact, capsaicin and its analogue capsinoids mimic the effects of cold to decrease body fatness through the activation and recruitment of BAT. The antiobesity effect of some other food ingredients, including

tea catechins, may also be attributable to the activation of the TRP-BAT axis. Thus, BAT is a promising target for combating obesity and related metabolic disorders in humans.[34]

- BAT is the site of sympathetically activated adaptive thermogenesis during cold exposure and after hyperphagia, thereby controlling whole-body energy expenditure and body fat. Cold-stimulated increase in glucose uptake is accompanied by a parallel increase in oxidative capacity, oxygen consumption, and blood flow in human BAT. In addition to stimulating activity, prolonged cooling increases BAT mass and induces browning of white adipose tissue in rodents.[35]
- BAT activity is reduced in the obese, and its stimulation by cold exposure increases insulin sensitivity and reduces body fat.[35]

Video Games

- Digital action games require sensory discrimination, leading to efficient and rapid information processing; they are adaptive, with increasingly difficult levels made available after achieving success at lower levels of performance, and are challenging and enjoyable.
- Twenty-three percent of individuals aged 65 years and older play digital games. Gamers aged 65 years and older play more frequently than any other age group, with 36% reporting play every day or nearly every day compared with 19% to 20% of gamers between 18 and 64 years of age. It is assumed that this is because gamers older than 65 years have more leisure time for play.[36]
- Engaging in cognitive activities, including those associated with digital action games, may potentially help older adults who do not develop dementia to improve or otherwise maintain cognitive abilities.[37]
- Action video game play may facilitate a general speed of processing improvement, presumably by the games' demands for fast and frequent decisions, the use of a dynamic display and a rich environment to explore, the need for divided attention at all times, and the rapid pace requiring nonstop decision-making.
- Active video games provide light-intensity exercise in community-dwelling older people, whether played while seated or standing. People who are unable to stand may derive equivalent benefits from active video games played while seated. The energy expenditure increases between 1.46 and 2.97 metabolic equivalent tasks when playing 5-minute bouts 9 times.[38] A meta-analysis also showed that active video games can also improve measures of mobility and balance in older people when used either on their own or as part of an exercise program.[39]
- There is as yet no evidence that using virtual reality games will prevent falls; but there is an indication that their use in balance training may improve balance control, which in turn may lead to falls prevention.

Sleep and Circadian Rhythms

- Daily rhythms of sleep and activity and the associated rhythms in metabolic states emerges from a complex interplay of endogenous cell autonomous circadian oscillators, daily exposure to light and darkness, and daily patterns of feeding and fasting.[40]
- The molecular clock reciprocally regulates the cells' internal environment, including redox state, nicotinamide adenine dinucleotide levels, energy state, and calcium levels.
- The circadian system is a master integrator of both the internal state of the organism and the organism interaction with nutrition and ambient light.

- Modern humans override the natural mechanism by self-selecting a sleep-wake pattern.
- The internal clock regulates inflammation by regulating expression of proinflammatory cytokines.
- Circadian systems modulate insulin and glucagon.
- Circadian disruptions have been shown to induce an intestinal microbial imbalance or maladaptation that can be restored by enforcing feeding-fasting patterns. It also increases risk of cancer, CVD, obesity, immune disorders, infertility, and affective and cognitive disorders
- In rodents, maintaining a regular daily feeding-fasting pattern may be sufficient to restore robust circadian rhythms to optimize physiology and decrease the risk of disease and increase health span.[40]
- Age-related diseases as well as aging can have adverse effects on the circadian clock. Mice fed a high-fat diet[41] along with time-restricted feeding during active periods are protected against obesity, hyperinsulinemia, hepatic steatosis, and inflammation with improvement of clock gene expression pattern. This finding suggests that maintaining circadian metabolic cycles can prevent age-related diseases and probably aging.

SUMMARY

Preventive measures are an indispensable part of promoting a healthier aging process. Careful attention to nutrition, environmental factors, and lifestyle, even though they will not prevent aging, could lead to a longer health span. Exercise is a very powerful promoter of health. As we age, more leisure time is available and the risk of a sedentary life increases. The author reviewed multiple activities that can be implemented safely during aging and added to regular endurance and strengthening exercises to promote a better QOL and a longer health span. Activities, such as meditation, yoga, TC, dancing, music, and others, can improve cognitive abilities, memory, and balance and decrease the risk of falls and maintain a more active lifestyle, maybe slowing some of the expected physical and cognitive deterioration. These activities can be done in groups and be modified for everybody to enjoy also providing a means to improve the social environment of the elderly with added benefits in mood, sleep, and QOL.

REFERENCES

1. Drewnowski A, Evans WJ. Nutrition, physical activity, and quality of life in older adults: summary. J Gerontol 2001;56A(11):89–94.
2. World Health Organization. Global recommendations on physical activity for health. 1. Exercise. 2. Life style. 3. Health promotion. 4. Chronic disease - prevention and control. 5. National health programs. Geneva (Switzerland): WHO; 2010.
3. Garber CE, Blissmer B, Deschenes MR, et al. Quantity and quality of exercise for developing and maintaining cardiorespiratory, musculoskeletal, and neuromotor fitness in apparently healthy adults: guidance for prescribing exercise. Med Sci Sports Exerc 2011;43(7):1334–59.
4. Paterson DH, Warburton DE. Physical activity and functional limitations in older adults: a systematic review related to Canada's physical activity guidelines. Int J Behav Nutr Phys Act 2010;7:38.
5. Edwards MK, Loprinzi PD. All-cause mortality risk as a function of sedentary behavior, moderate-to-vigorous physical activity and cardiorespiratory fitness. Phys Sportsmed 2016;44(3):223–30.

6. Mock JT, Chaudari K, Sidhu A, et al. The influence of vitamins E and C on brain aging. Exp Gerontol 2016;94:69–72.
7. Wayne PM, Manor B, Novak V, et al. A systems biology approach to studying tai chi, physiological complexity and healthy aging: design and rationale of a pragmatic randomized controlled trial. Contemp Clin trials 2013;34(1):21–34.
8. Taylor-Piliae RE, Newell KA, Cherin R, et al. Effects of tai chi and Western exercise on physical and cognitive functioning in healthy community-dwelling older adults. J Aging Phys Act 2010;18(3):261–79.
9. Huang Z-G, Feng Y-H, Li Y-H, et al. Systematic review and meta-analysis: tai chi for preventing falls in older adults. BMJ Open 2017;7(2):e013661.
10. Chan AW, Yu DS, Choi K, et al. Tai chi qigong as a means to improve night-time sleep quality among older adults with cognitive impairment: a pilot randomized controlled trial. Clin Interv Aging 2016;11:1277–86.
11. Wang XQ, Pi YL, Chen PJ, et al. Traditional Chinese exercise for cardiovascular diseases: systematic review and meta-analysis of randomized controlled trials. J Am Heart Assoc 2016;5:e002562.
12. Balaji PA, Varne SR, Ali SS. Physiological effects of yogic practices and transcendental meditation in health and disease. North Am J Med Sci 2012;4(10):442–8.
13. Manocha R, Marks GB, Kenchinton P, et al. Sahaja yoga in the management of moderate to severe asthma: a randomized controlled trial. Thorax 2002;57:110–5.
14. Bushell WC. Longevity: potential life span and health span enhancement through practice of the basic yoga meditation regimen. Ann N Y Acad Sci 2009;1172: 20–7.
15. Twal WO, Wahlquist AE, Balasubramanian S. Yogic breathing when compared to attention control reduces the levels of pro-inflammatory biomarkers in saliva: a pilot randomized controlled trial. BMC Complement Altern Med 2016;16:294.
16. Acevedo BP, Pospos S, Lavretsky H. The neural mechanisms of meditative practices: novel approaches for healthy aging. Curr Behav Neurosci Rep 2016;3(4): 328–39.
17. Goldin PR, Gross JJ. Effects of mindfulness-based stress reduction (mbsr) on emotion regulation in social anxiety disorder. Emotion 2010;10(1):83–91.
18. Dakwar E, Levin FR. Individual mindfulness-based psychotherapy for cannabis or cocaine dependence: a pilot feasibility trial. Am J Addict 2013;22(6):521–6.
19. Zeidan F, Martucci KT, Kraft RA, et al. Brain mechanisms supporting modulation of pain by mindfulness meditation. J Neurosci 2011;31(14):5540–8.
20. Marciniak R, Sheardova K, Čermáková P, et al. Effect of meditation on cognitive functions in context of aging and neurodegenerative diseases. Front Behav Neurosci 2014;8:17.
21. Verghese J, Lipton RB, Katz MJ, et al. Leisure activities and the risk of dementia in the elderly. N Engl J Med 2003;348:2508–16.
22. McNeely M, Duncan R, Earhart G. A comparison of dance interventions in people with Parkinson disease and older adults. Maturitas 2015;81(1):10–6.
23. Heiberger L, Maurer C, Amtage F, et al. Impact of a weekly dance class on the functional mobility and on the quality of life of individuals with Parkinson's disease. Front Aging Neurosci 2011;3:14.
24. Adam D, Ramli A, Shahar S. Effectiveness of a combined dance and relaxation intervention on reducing anxiety and depression and improving quality of life among the cognitively impaired elderly. Sultan Qaboos Univ Med J 2016;16(1): e47–53.

25. Marquez DX, Wilson R, Aguiñaga S, et al. Regular Latin dancing and health education may improve cognition of late middle-aged and older Latinos. J Aging Phys Act 2017;1–30. http://dx.doi.org/10.1123/japa.2016-0049.
26. Jia T, Ogawa Y, Miura M, et al. Music attenuated a decrease in parasympathetic nervous system activity after exercise. PLoS One 2016;11(2):e0148648.
27. Satoh M, Ogawa J, Tokita T, et al. The effects of physical exercise with music on cognitive function of elderly people: Mihama-Kiho Project. PLoS One 2014;9(4): e95230. Stam CJ, editor.
28. Levitin DJ, Chanda ML. The neurochemistry of music. Trends Cogn Sci 2013; 17(4):179–93.
29. Laukkanen T, Khan H, Zaccardi F, et al. Association between sauna bathing and fatal cardiovascular and all-cause mortality events. JAMA Intern Med 2015; 175(4):542–8.
30. Tamura Y, Kitaoka Y, Matsunaga Y, et al. Daily heat stress treatment rescues denervation-activated mitochondrial clearance and atrophy in skeletal muscle. J Physiol 2015;593(Pt 12):2707–20.
31. Littmann AE, Shields RK. Whole body heat stress increases motor cortical excitability and skill acquisition in humans. Clin Neurophysiol 2016;127(2):1521–9.
32. Chruściak T. Subjective evaluation of the effectiveness of whole-body cryotherapy in patients with osteoarthritis. Reumatologia 2016;54(6):291–5.
33. Hausswirth C, Schaal K, Le Meur Y, et al. Parasympathetic activity and blood catecholamine responses following a single partial-body cryostimulation and a whole-body cryostimulation. PLoS One 2013;8(8):e72658. Lucia A, editor.
34. Saito M, Yoneshiro T, Matsushita M. Activation and recruitment of brown adipose tissue by cold exposure and food ingredients in humans. Best Pract Res Clin Endocrinol Metab 2016;30(4):537–47.
35. Thuzar M, Ho KK. MECHANISMS IN ENDOCRINOLOGY: brown adipose tissue in humans: regulation and metabolic significance. Eur J Endocrinol 2016;175: R11–25.
36. Lenhart A, Jones S, Macgill AR. Pew internet project data memo. Pew Internet & AmericanLifeProject 2008. Available at: www.pewinternet.org/~/media//Files/Reports/2008/PIP_Adult_gaming_memo.pdf.pdf.
37. Zelinski EM, Reyes R. Cognitive benefits of computer games for older adults. Gerontechnology 2009;8(4):220–35.
38. Taylor LM, Maddison R. Activity and energy expenditure in older people playing active video games. Arch Phys Med Rehabil 2012;93(12):2281–6.
39. Taylor LM, Kerse N, Frakking T, et al. Active video games for improving physical performance measures in older people: a meta-analysis. J Geriatr Phys Ther 2016. [Epub ahead of print].
40. Manoogian EN, Panda S. Circadian rhythms, time restricted feeding, and healthy aging. Ageing Res Rev 2016. http://dx.doi.org/10.1016/j.arr.2016.12.006.
41. Nakahata Y, Bessho Y. The circadian NAD^+ metabolism: impact on chromatin remodeling and aging. Biomed Res Int 2016;2016:3208429.

Can We Increase Our Health Span?

Carlos E. Rivera-Tavarez, MD

KEYWORDS

• Aging • Health span • Inflammation • Chronic disease • Lifestyle

KEY POINTS

- The deterioration of physical and mental capabilities is inevitable with aging.
- Even though some hereditary factors cannot be changed, many other external factors can be manipulated to provide our body with better weapons to have a better quality of life as we age.
- Different cellular pathways that lead to cell deterioration and aging usually act through excessive oxidative damage and chronic inflammation.
- Suppression of inflammation is the most important driver of successful longevity and increases in importance with advancing age.
- Lower inflammation is associated with prolonged physical functionality and cognitive abilities.

Aging brings a cascade of ills and health problems leading to the deterioration of physical, mental, emotional, and social dimensions of life.[1] It is influenced by hereditary and environmental factors. The hereditary factors, like physical and mental abilities, will inevitably deteriorate, but the external, environmental factors like level of physical activity, nutrition, and lifestyle can be controlled and regulated.[1] Life expectancy has been increasing and is projected to continue this trend and reach more than 80 years in most industrialized countries by 2030 with some reaching up to 90 years.[2] As important and exciting as this is, an increased lifespan without corresponding quality of life may not be very meaningful. In this article, we review the theories of aging, some of its physiologic processes, and possible ways to increase our health span and decrease morbidity by limiting progression or development of some of the most common risks of aging, including cardiovascular diseases, diabetes, cerebrovascular disorders, cancer, and neurodegenerative disorders.

The author has nothing to disclose.
Campbell Clinic Orthopedics, 1211 Union Avenue, Memphis, TN 38104, USA
E-mail address: crivera@campbellclinic.com

Phys Med Rehabil Clin N Am 28 (2017) 681–692
http://dx.doi.org/10.1016/j.pmr.2017.08.002
1047-9651/17/© 2017 Elsevier Inc. All rights reserved.

pmr.theclinics.com

THEORIES OF AGING

There are different theories and factors to try to explain aging and its changes, although it is well understood that it is a multifactorial process.[3] Some of these will follow.

1. Wear and tear: compares humans to machines. Accumulation of excessive consumption of fat, sugar, and UV radiation will cause cell damage and death. Disregards the cell capacity for self-repair.
2. Stochastic theory sees aging as the result of inevitable, random, small changes that accumulate over time.
3. Evolutionary theory: Specific genes are implicated in longevity and in maintenance of the cells. These genes are susceptible to mutations with age.
4. Rate of living theory: organisms that metabolize oxygen more rapidly have a higher energy expenditure and shorter lifespan.
5. Oxidative stress theory: most frequently cited lately and possibly the most important one with regard to increasing health span. Age-associated functional losses are due to the accrual of oxidative damage to macromolecules, such as lipids, DNA, proteins by free radicals, and that the progressive oxidant/antioxidant imbalance leads to the consequent disruption of redox-regulated signaling mechanisms.

CAUSES OF AGING

1. Failure of cellular metabolism, decreasing secretion of body hormones, and environmental factors, such as quality of diet, lack of physical activity. Discrepancy between biological damage and the rate of repair leads to accumulation of damage, especially through oxidation.[1]
2. Cell determinants of aging include free radical damage, mitochondrial dysfunction, decreased autophagy, alterations of glucose and cholesterol metabolism, telomere shortening, and increased apoptosis[4]
3. Mitochondria dysfunction.
   - Mitochondria are responsible for most of the useful energy derived from the breakdown of carbohydrates and fatty acids, which are converted to ATP by the process of oxidative phosphorylation.
   - Mitochondria are a major source of reactive oxygen species (ROS) and reactive nitrogen species (RNS) that can regulate mitochondrial activity through different mechanisms, including modulation of O_2 consumption and oxidative phosphorylation, induction of mitochondrial membrane permeability transition, regulation of mitochondrial biogenesis, mitochondrial dynamics, and autophagy/mitophagy.[5]
     - Excessive ROS production is usually compensated by the antioxidant defense system, thus maintaining the redox balance. Cellular antioxidants, including enzymes, such as superoxide dismutase and catalase (CAT) and low-molecular-weight antioxidants, such as vitamins C and E, and glutathione peroxidase (GPX), are the main orchestrators of this defensive barrier.
   - Mitochondria are a primary target of the aging process, as evidenced by a decline in mitochondrial oxidative capacity in both skeletal and heart muscle with age.
     - Aging has been associated with excessive oxidative stress and overproduction of RNS. Indeed, oxidative/nitrosative stress is thought to be an important contributor to the degeneration of long-lived post-mitotic cells, such as cardiomyocytes and neurons. This explains in part the relation between acquired cardiac and neurodegenerative diseases and aging.

- Factors affecting mitochondrial biogenesis:
  - It is well established that physical activity increases mitochondrial content.
  - Peroxisome proliferator-activated receptor gamma coactivator 1-alpha (PGC-1α) is a protein and a major regulator of mitochondrial biogenesis.
    - Cold, exercise, and electrical stimulation can promote it.
    - PGC-1α plays a crucial role in linking stimuli, such as cold or exercise, to an internal metabolic response like mitochondrial biogenesis via, among others, the nuclear respiratory factor (NRF) transcription factors.
  - Amp-activated protein kinase (AMPK) is an enzyme that works as a major regulator of mitochondrial biogenesis controlling intracellular energy metabolism in response to acute energy crises.
    - AMPK activity is reduced with aging and that it may be an important contributing factor in mitochondrial dysfunction and dysregulated intracellular lipid metabolism.
  - Nitric oxide (NO), Sirtuin 1, and Calcineurin are also associated to mitochondrial biogenesis.
    - Calcineurin is a calcium/calmodulin-dependent protein phosphatase known to be the master regulator of fast-to-slow twitch muscle fiber–type changes.
  - Mitochondrial antioxidant treatments:
    - Exercise-induced ROS generation reduces insulin resistance and causes an adaptive response by which the endogenous antioxidant defense capacity is enhanced. Thus, supplementation with antioxidants may preclude the health-promoting effects of exercise in humans.
    - Metallothioneins
      - Proteins in the membrane of the Golgi apparatus that play important roles in many biological processes, such as metal ion homeostasis and detoxification, protection of cells from oxidative stress, cell proliferation, and cell survival. Their expression can be induced by many stimuli, including hormones, cytokines, metal ions, and oxidating agents.

4. Apoptosis
   - The process of cell suicide when a cell is no longer needed. It involves many cells, even healthy ones. Cells die neatly without causing inflammation or damage to the neighbors. They shrink, condense, and then are phagocytosed by macrophages.[6]
   - Apoptosis also occurs as a defense mechanism, such as in immune reactions or when cells are damaged by disease or noxious agents.
   - Inappropriate apoptosis (either too little or too much) is a factor in many human conditions, including neurodegenerative diseases, ischemic damage, autoimmune disorders, and many types of cancer.[7]

5. Cellular senescence
   - Cellular senescences are the tumor-constraining mechanisms that halt the proliferation of cells after a finite number of population doublings, allowing the organism to antagonize the potentially detrimental effects of uncontrolled growth.
   - Usually triggered by telomere shortening.[3] A DNA damage response (DDR), triggered by uncapped telomeres or nontelomeric DNA damage, is the most prominent initiator of senescence.
   - ROSs are likely to be involved in establishment and stabilization of senescence; elevated ROS levels are associated with both replicative (telomere-dependent) and stress-induced or oncogene-induced senescence. Mitochondrial dysfunction and ROS production can not only accelerate the onset of senescence (eg, by accelerating telomere shortening), but are also components and a

consequence of continuous DDR signaling and are thus an integral part of the senescent phenotype.[8]

- Irreversible senescence-associated secretory phenotype can promote diseases by perpetuating a proinflammatory state.
- Declining mitochondrial function and biogenesis along with increased systemic inflammation and decreased growth factor (GF) levels with aging leads to apoptosis and senescence.

6. Telomeres[9]

- Repeating segments of noncoding DNA at the ends of the chromosomes. They shorten with each cell division and help determine how fast cells age and when they die.
- Short telomeres in aged cells may be recognized as DNA double-strand breaks, ultimately causing the cell to enter senescence. Cells with short telomeres send out constant inflammatory signals.
- Telomerase: enzyme responsible for restoring the DNA lost during cell division. Makes and replenishes telomeres.
- Telomere length can be altered by the following:
  o Psychological stress (depression, anxiety, pessimism) decreases telomerase and telomere length.
  o Meditation, chanting, and deep restoration techniques that reduce stress stimulate telomerase.
  o Exercise
    ▪ Cherkas and colleagues[10] reported a positive association between increasing physical activity and longer telomeres, with differences in telomere length equating to approximately 10 years of biological age difference between active and inactive subjects.
    ▪ Moderate aerobic endurance and high-intensity interval training have been better than resistance exercises. Regardless of exercise, those who increase their aerobic fitness have greater telomerase activity.
    ▪ Extreme exercise (ultra-marathons) is not better than ordinary levels of exercise, but overtraining damages telomeres.
  o People who sleep at least 7 hours have longer telomeres.
  o TA-65MD
    ▪ This is a patented compound that was discovered as a chemically defined small molecule activator of telomerase from an empirical screen of natural product extracts of traditional Chinese medicines.
    ▪ Without telomerase, telomeres gradually shorten with each cell division due to the end replication problem, oxidative stress, and other natural DNA processing at chromosome ends, ultimately triggering cell senescence and ensuing tissue degeneration when telomeres become critically short.[11]
    ▪ A randomized, double-blind, placebo-controlled study on healthy cytomegalovirus-positive people showed that 250U of TA-65MD over 12 months increased telomere length compared with placebo and high doses of the compound(1000U).[12]

7. Autophagy
  o Autophagy is a general term for the degradation of cytoplasmic components within lysosomes.
  o However, recent studies have clearly demonstrated that autophagy has a greater variety of physiologic and pathophysiological roles than expected, such as starvation adaptation, intracellular protein and organelle clearance, development,

antiaging, elimination of microorganisms, cell death, tumor suppression, and antigen presentation.[13]

o Autophagy is a self-degradative process that is important for balancing sources of energy at critical times in development and in response to nutrient stress. Autophagy also plays a housekeeping role in removing misfolded or aggregated proteins, clearing damaged organelles, such as mitochondria, endoplasmic reticulum, and peroxisomes, as well as eliminating intracellular pathogens. Thus, autophagy is generally thought of as a survival mechanism, although its deregulation has been linked to nonapoptotic cell death.[14]

GENETIC INFLUENCE

Although it is very difficult to prove that a gene influences aging in humans, a relationship may be inferred based on whether a genetic variant is found more frequently among successful agers compared with a group of people who have an average or short lifespan. Most longevity genes thus far influence 1 of 3 pathways in a cell: sirtuins, mechanistic target of rapamycin (mTOR), and insulin/insulin like growth factor-1 (IGF-1).

Sirtuins

- Class of proteins that regulate key cellular processes, such as cell cycle, apoptosis, metabolic regulation, and inflammation.[15] These proteins decrease with aging and are implicated in a wide spectrum of diseases like cancer, diabetes type 2, obesity, neurodegenerative disorders, and longevity. They require beta nicotinamide adenine dinucleotide (NAD+) as a co-substrate.
- Studies have reported changes in expression of SIRT1 and activity linked to mitochondrial function alterations following hypoxic ischemic conditions and following reoxygenation injury.
- Aging decreases tissue levels of NAD, decreasing sirtuin activity and decreasing NAD/NADH leading to an increase in ROS.
- SIRT1
  o Regulates apoptosis inhibition of P53 (tumor suppressor gene) and DNA repair.
  o Regulates neurogenesis and mitochondrial biogenesis.
  o Controls inflammatory regulator NF-kB.
  o Inhibits NO, ROS.
  o Tumor suppressor.
  o Maintains lipid homeostasis; during fasting mobilizes fat from white adipose tissue (WAT).
  o Controls mitochondrial biogenesis regulating PGC-1.
  o Regulates AMPK.
  o Upregulates insulin secretion.
  o Helps maintain circadian rhythms.
- SIRT2, among other things, activates autophagy.
- SIRT3
  o Essential for the caloric restriction (CR)-mediated mitigation of oxidative damage by regulating the glutathione antioxidant system, thereby regulating senescence-associated pathologies propagated by oxidative stress.[3]

Mechanistic or Mammalian Target of Rapamycin

- An enzyme that has a role in mediating nutrient signaling, autophagy, and growth regulation.[3]

- o Also regulates cell survival and spatial organization of the cytoskeleton.
- o Autophagy is increased by amino acid or glucose deprivation or decreased insulin.
- Inhibition of mTOR by rapamycin.
  - o Counter damage inducing senescence mechanisms and enhancing repair pathways resulting in extended lifespan.
- Inhibited by cellular stress (hypoxia), low energy.
- Responsive to growth factors.
- Increased activity by excess nutrients leads to increase oxidative stress by enhancing mitochondrial consumption.

FOXO3 GENE

- A strong association between FOXO3 and longevity has been reported in long lived American men of Japanese ancestry[16,17]
- Along with Apolipoprotein E, one of the only 2 genes that have been replicated consistently across diverse human populations for association with extreme old age.
- It is stimulated by stress (especially oxidative), and declines during aging. Promotes gluconeogenesis, DNA repair, cell cycle arrest, stem cell homeostasis (primary driver in humans), and immune system modulation; increases apoptosis, redox balance, breaks down ROS, lipophagy, mitophagy, and proteostasis.
- Implicated in insulin/IGF-1 signaling, decreasing its activity.
- Suppresses members of the mTOR pathway.
- Immune system
  - o Controls cytokine production, opposes nuclear factor kappa-light-chain-enhancer of activated B cells (NF-kB) activation, suppresses T-cell activation and proliferation, decreases proliferation of lymphatic cells, and lowers inflammation.
  - o Counters toxic protein aggregation seeing in neurodegenerative disorders.
  - o Suppresses tumor growth.
- Protects against Diabetes Mellitus type 2 (DM2) cardiovascular diseases, cancer, neurodegenerative disorders.

Caloric Restriction

- Limiting total energy intake 10% to 40% less than ad libitum, while maintaining enough intake of nutrients and vitamins.
- CR is the only nongenetic and the most consistently successful nonpharmacological intervention extending lifespan in organisms from yeast to mammals.[4] It is the most profound method for reducing the aging process.[1,18]
- CR increase in health span is inversely related to amount of CR and positively related to the duration of the restriction.[19]
- Okinawans, predominantly vegetarian, consume approximately 80% of calories than the rest of Japan, have more centenarians per million, and the lowest death rate from cardiovascular disease and stroke than any other population.[20]

Effects of caloric restriction

- Decreases body weight (BW), body fat, C-reactive protein, triglycerides, low-density lipoprotein, cholesterol:high-density lipoprotein ratio.[4]

- Increases whole body energy efficiency by inducing the biogenesis of mitochondria that use less oxygen and produce fewer ROS.
- Increases glucose tolerance and insulin sensitivity.
- Increases anti-inflammatory hormones like adiponectin, ghrelin, corticosterone.
  - Chronic inflammation is often associated with tissue injury, increased fibrosis, and organ dysfunction, and is involved in the pathogenesis of many age-related diseases and in the aging process itself.
- Decreases anabolic hormones: IGF-1, insulin, testosterone (T), leptin, estradiol, and growth hormone (GH)/IGF-1 axis.
  - In rodents, decreased IGF-1 is related to longevity.
- Modulates cell survival and apoptosis and stimulates autophagy.
- Remodels WAT, lowering proinflammatory adipokine and cytokine levels and decreasing oxidative stress.
- Enhances expression of heat shock proteins.
- Stimulates hormesis.
  - Process in which chronic low stress elicits a defensive response that helps protect against other, stronger, subsequent stressors, thus favoring enhanced longevity.
- Regulates metabolism of Peroxisome PGC-1α, AMPK, IGF-1, and mTOR.
  a. PGC-1α
     - Protects against the decline in mitochondrial function characteristic of skeletal muscle aging.
     - Protects against the age-induced metabolic shift in the heart from lipid to cholesterol metabolism.
     - Protects against the age-related alteration of adipose tissue distribution and function.
     - Induces the expression of genes involved in the mitochondrial electron transport system.
     - Increases mitochondrial biogenesis.
  b. AMPK
     - Activated in response to an increase in the intracellular AMP/ATP ratio.
     - Increases fatty acid oxidation.
     - Increases autophagy.
     - Increases insulin sensitivity and glucose uptake by muscle decreasing blood glucose levels.
     - Decreases glucose absorption in the gastrointestinal tract.
     - Inhibits gluconeogenesis in liver.
     - Downregulates IGF-1 therefore, activates FOXO that induces transcription of antioxidant genes.
       - Suppresses cyclooxygenase (COX)-derived reactive species generation.[21]
         - COX is responsible for the formation of prostaglandins, prostacyclin, and thromboxane.
         - By decreasing thromboxane 2, prostaglandin E2 and prostacyclin stimulates NF-kB activity.
         - NF-kB is responsible for the transcription of many proinflammatory proteins like tumor necrosis factor (TNF)-alpha, interleukin (IL)1, IL2, IL6, COX2, nitric oxide synthase.
       - Decreases age-related inflammation and proinflammatory cytokine production in humans.[21]
       - Increases expression of SIRT1 that inhibits NF-kB, blocking production of inflammatory mediators.

Caloric restriction mimetics

- Main problem with CR is that it is very difficult to maintain for long periods.[1] Therefore, any substance that can simulate or replicate some of the effects of CR can have benefits in improving health span and is worth evaluating. These substances are called caloric restriction mimetics (CRMs).
- Ideally should reproduce the metabolic, hormonal, and physiologic effects of CR, activate stress response pathways similar to CR, produce CR-like effects on mortality and age-related disease, and induce no significant reduction in long-term food consumption.[4,22]
- CRM targeting glucose metabolism[19]
  1. Glycolytic inhibitors decrease cell use of glucose.
     - 2-deoxyglucose
       ○ Glucose analog that is taken by cells but not further metabolized, competitively inhibits glucose utilization thus resulting in decreased energy production.[4]
  2. Insulin sensitizers
     - Thiazolidinediones: pioglitazone/rosiglitazone[23]
       ○ Activators of the peroxisome proliferator-activated receptors.
       ○ Pioglitazone has been shown to induce mitochondrial biogenesis by the activation of the PGC-1α pathway in human subcutaneous adipose tissue.
       ○ Rosiglitazone treatment for 8 weeks also increased expression of PGC-1α and activity of oxidative enzymes in skeletal muscle of patients with type 2 diabetes.
  3. Metformin
     - A growing body of evidence from clinical studies and animal models suggests that the primary function of metformin is to decrease hepatic glucose production, mainly by inhibiting gluconeogenesis.[24]
     - Multiple pathways but the better known one is the activation of cellular energy regulatory sensor AMPK.
     - Has also been shown to increase the skeletal muscle content of PGC-1α in rats, suggesting increased mitochondrial biogenesis.
  4. Acarbose/Precose
     - When consumed with complex carbohydrate (CHO) meals
       ○ Is a competitive inhibitor of CHO breakdown along brush border of the small intestine.
       ○ Has 15,000 times more affinity than sucrose for glucosidase that reduces the enzymatic degradation and absorption of glucose from complex CHOs.
       ○ Lowers postprandial glucose, HbA1c, and BW in humans.
       ○ Increases lifespan in mice.
  5. Na/Gly cotransporter 2 inhibitors
     - Increase clearance of blood glucose.
     - Decrease recovery of glucose from glomerular filtrate increasing glucose excretion.
  6. Resistant starches
     - Increase fermentation in gut and decrease rate of colon cancer, CHO, and blood glucose.
  7. Short-chain fatty acids
     - Important to decrease inflammation.

- Main source in body is from byproducts of carbohydrate fermentation in gut.
  - Colon epithelial cells can use it as fuel or absorb it into blood.
  - Activates suppressors of inflammation.
8. Other glucosidase or amylase inhibitors
   - Leguminous plants
   - Cinnamon: It helps lower blood sugar levels and also can improve sensitivity to insulin. Blocks enzymes called alanines, which allows for glucose to be absorbed into the blood. Therefore, it has been shown to decrease the amount of glucose that enters the bloodstream after a high-sugar meal.
   - Sweet potatoes
9. SIRT1 activating compounds (STACS)
   - Resveratrol
     - Abundant in grapes: Protects neurons against mutant glutamine toxicity. Also, may improve insulin sensitivity and promotes autophagy by activating NAD-dependent SIRT1.
     - Most potent of the natural activators has been shown to inhibit the activity and expression of NADPH oxidase in cardiovascular tissues, to accelerate mitochondrial ROS detoxification by upregulating SOD2, and to reduce mitochondrial radical production.
     - It can also decrease insulin and glucose levels, enhance mitochondrial function, and suppress inflammation in healthy obese men. Its beneficial effects have also been demonstrated in type 2 diabetes by decreasing cholesterol, blood pressure, and HbA1c levels, while it promoted insulin sensitivity in the elderly
     - It can cross the blood–brain barrier and reach the brain tissue rapidly after systemic administration, an effect related to the therapeutic potential of this compound in stroke and neurodegenerative diseases.
   - Polyphenols
     - Abundant in green tea.
       - Catechin has been reported to modulate and energy-intensive stress response and repair system.
       - Epicatechin (also abundant in cocoa) reduces inflammatory markers, increases antioxidant defenses and improves AMPK.
     - Apples and blueberries are also great sources.
   - Curcumin
     - May delay cell senescence.
     - Also has an effect on TOR pathways; therefore, possible anticancer effects.
     - It is a powerful antioxidant and anti-inflammatory.
10. Nonpolyphenol STACS
    - Omega 3 fatty acid
      - Improves cardiovascular health
      - Improves autoimmune disorders
      - Improves neurodegenerative disorders
    - Melatonin
      - Improves pro-survival signals and reduces pro-death signals in mice.
11. Lipoic acid
    - Potent antioxidant and mitochondrial metabolite, stimulates glutathione synthesis, enhances insulin signaling, and modulates the activity of other cell-signaling molecules and transcription factors.

- Associated with improvement of age-associated cognitive dysfunction of brain in rats, dogs,[25] and humans.[26]
- Improves vascular endothelial cell function, decreases inflammation, ameliorates lipid abnormalities, and protects against myocardial ischemia/reperfusion injury or antihypertensive effects.

12. Epigallocatechin gallate[27]

Extends lifespan in healthy rats by reducing liver and kidney damage and improving age-associated inflammation and oxidative stress through the inhibition of NF-kB signaling by activating the longevity factors FOXO3 and SIRT1.

Most abundant catechin in tea (green > white > black).

Also in small amounts in apple skin, plums, onions, hazelnuts, and pecans.

13. CoQ10

Persson and colleagues[28] demonstrated restored mitochondrial O_2 consumption and an improvement in mitochondrial and renal functions in diabetic mice fed a diet supplemented with CoQ10.

Because CoQ10 is present at high concentrations in the heart, its potential benefits for cardiac dysfunction have been widely tested in humans with discrepant results.

14. Mito Q

Is the most extensively evaluated and best-understood mitochondria-targeted antioxidant. Mito Q uptake occurs primarily in mitochondria rather than in other cell compartments.

Escribano-Lopez and colleagues[29] showed that it has an anti-inflammatory and antioxidant action in the leukocytes of patients with type 2 diabetes mellitus by decreasing ROS production, leukocyte-endothelium interactions, and TNF-α through the action of NFκB. The long-term administration of mitochondria-targeted mitoquinone mesylate failed to attenuate age-related oxidative damage in skeletal muscle of old mice or provide any protective effect in the context of muscle aging.[30]

15. Ursolic acid

- The major waxy component in apple peels.
- Reduces skeletal muscle atrophy in the setting of 2 distinct atrophies.
- Inducing stresses (fasting and muscle denervation).
- Can induce muscle hypertrophy by enhancing skeletal muscle insulin/IGF-I signaling, and inhibiting atrophy-associated skeletal muscle mRNA expression.
- Importantly, effects on muscle were accompanied by reductions in adiposity, fasting blood glucose, and plasma cholesterol and triglycerides. These findings identify a potential therapy for muscle atrophy and perhaps other metabolic diseases.[31,32]

SUMMARY

The deterioration of physical and mental capabilities is inevitable with aging. Even though some hereditary factors cannot be changed, many other external factors can be manipulated to provide our body with better weapons to have a better quality of life as we age. Different cellular pathways that lead to cell deterioration and aging usually act through excessive oxidative damage and chronic inflammation. Suppression of inflammation is the most important driver of successful longevity and increases in importance with advancing age. Lower inflammation is associated with prolonged physical functionality and cognitive abilities. Modifications of our caloric intake, amount and type of food, as well as maintaining an active lifestyle can lead to maintenance of our antioxidative, anti-inflammatory pathways and decrease the risk of the most common chronic diseases of aging that bring most of the age-related diseases, like cardiovascular diseases, diabetes, cancer, and neurodegenerative conditions.

REFERENCES

1. Bhar GC. In search of rationality in human longevity and immortality. Mens Sana Monogr 2016;14:187–213.
2. Kontis V, Bennett JE, Mathers CD, et al. Future life expectancy in 35 industrialised countries: projections with a Bayesian model ensemble. Lancet 2017;389(10076): 1323–35.
3. Chandrasekaran A, Idelchik MDPS, Melendez JA. Redox control of senescence and age-related disease. Redox Biol 2017;11:91–102.
4. Testa G, Biasi F, Poli G, et al. Calorie restriction and dietary restriction mimetics: a strategy for improving healthy aging and longevity. Curr Pharm Des 2014;20: 2950–77.
5. Apostolova N, Victor VM. Molecular strategies for targeting antioxidants to mitochondria: therapeutic implications. Antioxid Redox Signal 2015;22:686–729.
6. Alberts B, Johnson A, Lewis J. Molecular biology of the cell. 4th edition. New York: Garland Science; 2002.
7. Elmore S. Apoptosis: a review of programmed cell death. Toxicol Pathol 2007;35: 495–516.
8. Passos JF, Nelson G, Wang C, et al. Feedback between p21 and reactive oxygen production is necessary for cell senescence. Mol Syst Biol 2010;6:347.
9. Blackburn E, Epel E. The telomere effect: a revolutionary approach to living younger, healthier, longer. New York: Grand Central Publushing. Hachette Book Group; 2017.
10. Cherkas LF, Hunkin JL, Kato BS, et al. The association between physical activity in leisure time and leukocyte telomere length. Arch Intern Med 2008;168:154–8.
11. Vaziri H, Dragowska W, Allsopp RC, et al. Evidence for a mitotic clock in human hematopoietic stem cells: loss of telomeric DNA with age. Proc Natl Acad Sci U S A 1994;91:9857–60.
12. Salvador L, Singaravelu G, Harley CB, et al. A natural product telomerase activator lengthens telomeres in humans: a randomized, double blind, and placebo controlled study. Rejuvenation Res 2016;19:478–84.
13. Mizushima N. Autophagy: process and function. Genes Dev 2007;21:2861–73.
14. Glick D, Barth S, Macleod KF. Autophagy: cellular and molecular mechanisms. J Pathol 2010;221:3–12.
15. Poulose N, Raju R. Sirtuin regulation in aging and injury. Biochim Biophys Acta 2015;1852:2442–55.
16. Morris BJ, Willcox DC, Donlon TA, et al. FOXO3: a major gene for human longevity—a mini-review. Gerontology 2015;61:515–25.
17. Bao JM, Song XL, Hong YQ, et al. Association between FOXO3A gene polymorphisms and human longevity: a meta-analysis. Asian J Androl 2014;16:446–52.
18. Rockenfeller P, Madeo F. Ageing and eating. Biochim Biophys Acta 2010;1803: 499–506.

19. Brewer RA, Gibbs VK, Smith DL Jr. Targeting glucose metabolism for healthy aging. Nutr Healthy Aging 2016;4:31–46.
20. Willcox DC, Willcox BJ, He Q. They really are that old: a validation study of centenarian prevalence in Okinawa. J Gerontol A Biol Sci Med Sci 2008;63A(4): 338–49.
21. Chung KW, Kim DH, Park MH, et al. Recent advances in calorie restriction research on aging. Exp Gerontol 2013;48:1049–53.
22. Ingram DK, Zhu M, Mamczarz J, et al. Calorie restriction mimetics: an emerging research field. Aging Cell 2006;5:97–108.
23. Jornayvaz FR, Shulman GI. Regulation of mitochondrial biogenesis. Essays Biochem 2010;47:69–84.
24. Benoit V, Guigas B. Cellular and molecular mechanisms of metformin: an overview. Clin Sci (Lond) 2012;122(6):253–70.
25. Aggarwal BB, Gupta SC, Sung B. Curcumin: an orally bioavailable blocker of TNF and other pro-inflammatory biomarkers. Br J Pharmacol 2013;169:1672–92.
26. Valk EE, Hornstra G. Relationship between vitamin E requirement and polyunsaturated fatty acid intake in man: a review. Int J Vitam Nutr Res 2000;70:31–42.
27. Niu Y, Na L. The phytochemical EGCG extends lifespan by reducing liver and kidney function damage and improving age-associated inflammation and oxidative stress in healthy rats. Aging Cell 2013;12:1041–9.
28. Persson MF, Franzén S, Catrina SB, et al. Coenzyme Q10 prevents GDP-sensitive mitochondrial uncoupling, glomerular hyperfiltration and proteinuria in kidneys from db/db mice as a model of type 2 diabetes. Diabetologia 2012;55:1535–43.
29. Escribano-Lopez I, Diaz-Morales N, Rovira-Llopis S, et al. The mitochondria-targeted antioxidant MitoQ modulates oxidative stress, inflammation and leukocyte-endothelium interactions in leukocytes isolated from type 2 diabetic patients. Redox Biol 2016;10:200–5.
30. Sakellariou GK, Pearson T, Lightfoot AP, et al. Long-term administration of the mitochondria-targeted antioxidant mitoquinone mesylate fails to attenuate age-related oxidative damage or rescue the loss of muscle mass and function associated with aging of skeletal muscle. FASEB J 2016;30:3771–85.
31. Kunkel SD, Suneja M, Ebert SM, et al. mRNA expression signatures of human skeletal muscle atrophy identify a natural compound that increases muscle mass. Cell Metab 2011;13:627–38.
32. Maggio M, Lauretani F, Ceda GP, et al. Relationship between low levels of anabolic hormones and 6-year mortality in older men: the aging in the Chianti Area (InCHIANTI) study. Arch Intern Med 2007;167:2249–54.

Psychosocial Issues in Geriatric Rehabilitation

Ricardo M. Rodriguez, PhD

KEYWORDS

- Geriatric • Psychosocial • Depression • Anxiety • Dementia • Adjustment
- Rehabilitation

KEY POINTS

- Identification and management of psychosocial issues commonly present in geriatric patients undergoing rehabilitation can help maximize gains and foster well-being.
- Interventions to address these issues can be carried out not only by mental health providers but also by rehabilitation staff in interdisciplinary teams to potentiate the effectiveness of interventions.
- Promoting a healthy perspective on aging and fostering resilience can have a positive impact during the rehabilitation process.
- Comprehensive assessment of geriatric patients is deemed to be essential to identify important areas of concern, risks, strengths and needs and to plan treatment accordingly.

INTRODUCTION

Efforts to achieve successful rehabilitation of individuals during late adulthood must account for a myriad of factors beyond medical conditions, mobility, and functional status. Psychological, cognitive, and social factors present challenges for rehabilitation specialists as they work toward recovery goals. Ignoring such factors can result in poor outcomes, increased health care costs, and frustration among providers. On the other hand, taking the time to identify, consider, and address these important aspects can help not only achieve rehabilitation goals but also improve quality of life for the older adult. This article focuses on briefly describing a selection of these factors, reviewing useful screening tools, and introducing strategies that can help the rehabilitation professional in multiple settings overcome these challenges and promote wellness as a goal. Finally, a focus on reinforcing personal strengths and promoting resilience in late adulthood is presented as an effective way of helping individuals cope and succeed at the task of aging in late adulthood.

Disclosure statement: The author has nothing to disclose.
Physical Medicine and Rehabilitation Service, VA Caribbean Health Care System, 10 Casia Street, San Juan, PR 00921, USA
E-mail address: Ricardo.Rodriguez-Medina@va.gov

DISCUSSION
Depression in Geriatric Patients

Aging is continuous process of change, which for many represents an opportunity to continue learning, share wisdom with others, and explore new goals. However, for others it can be seen as a time to experience an inevitable loss of abilities, function, roles, and often times loved ones. Mood, adjustment, and quality of life will depend greatly on these perspectives. Depression in response to the multiple stressors of late adulthood is well documented in the literature.[1] Prevalence rates of major depressive disorder among older adults, although lower than the younger populations, increase among those with medical conditions and those who are institutionalized.[1] Depression in geriatric patients can also be observed after disabling illnesses, such as stroke[2,3] and limb amputation.[4] Depressed patients can have increased risk of negative consequences, such as recurrent stroke and reduction in quality of life.[5] Increased health care costs have also been associated with depression.[5] Conversely, effective management of depression can have a positive impact on rehabilitation outcomes. For example, there is research suggesting that older patients whose depression is treated describe improvement in pain levels.[6] Rehabilitation providers and teams often become frustrated when patients with potential fail to benefit from interventions because of depressive symptoms. Being able to identify and manage geriatric patients with depression is deemed to be essential in achieving their rehabilitation goals.

Screening for depression in late adulthood

The presentation of depression in late adulthood may vary and requires understanding of particular issues of the population. A depressed older adult may not report depressed mood but evidence other symptoms.[7] At times, it might also be difficult to differentiate the mood disorder from medications side effects, impact of multiple comorbidities, and the effects of insomnia or fatigue. Somatic symptoms of depression may also be confounded with comorbid conditions commonly present in late adulthood. Relying on the criteria of the *Diagnostic and Statistical Manual of Mental Disorders*, Fifth Edition (*DSM-5*) for major depressive disorder will be of help but is not always sufficient. Exploring these symptoms further during an office visit, inpatient round, or consultation can yield important information that can make a significant impact in rehabilitation outcomes. A referral to a mental health provider may be appropriate and necessary, but detection and crafting a rehabilitation care plan based on findings are tasks that rest on rehabilitation staff.

Geriatric patients may minimize symptoms because of the stigma of mental illness or perceptions that depression may reflect weakness. However, for some, a questionnaire has the effect of normalizing symptoms suggesting that others may be experiencing what they are experiencing. Multiple, easy-to-administer screening tools exist that have been found to be valid among the elderly (**Table 1**).

The Geriatric Depression Scale in its 15-item version is designed to assess depression in late adulthood.[8] It relies less on somatic symptoms, emphasizing symptoms more frequently observed in older adults. Its format of yes/no responses can help reduce minimization of symptoms given its forced choice response options. This format can also be simpler for patients with cognitive impairment.[9,10] The Patient Health Questionnaire 9 item has been found to be a valid tool for detecting depression among those 65 years and older.[9] This measure is a self-report, 9-item questionnaire that can be completed in a short period of time. The measure also includes an item that assesses for self-harm ideas or death wishes, which if positive can open the door for further assessment and intervention. It is also a useful measure for tracking

Table 1 Screening tools for geriatric patients	
Assessment Domain	**Screening Test/Measure**
Depression	Geriatric Depression Scale (GDS)
	Patient Health Questionnaire (PHQ-9)
	Stroke Aphasia Depression Questionnaire
Anxiety	Geriatric Anxiety Scale
Neurocognitive screening	Mini-Mental State Examination (MMSE)
	Cognistat
	Montreal Cognitive Assessment (MoCA)
Caregiver burnout	Zarit Burden Scale

symptom severity because of its ease of use. In special populations, such as the individual with aphasia after stroke, the Stroke Aphasia Depression Questionnaire[11] can be a helpful tool for detecting and monitoring depression. This scale relies on staff observations of behaviors and ratings based on severity.

These instruments and other similar ones are not diagnostic. Further evaluation by a clinician is required to clarify responses or ask additional questions. For example, patients with a stroke may report not eating because of difficulty adapting to a dysphagia diet or simply because of a dislike of hospital food. Hospitalized patients may report not sleeping because of interruptions by staff at night. Patients may report crying spells or even death wishes in the context of acute pain experience. Further questioning is necessary to clarify responses and diagnosis. Ruling out other factors, such as thyroid problems, polypharmacy, effect of pain/anxiety medications, and other conditions that may mimic depression, is essential for an accurate diagnosis.

Interventions strategies

Use of selective serotonin reuptake inhibitors, psychotherapeutic modalities, such as cognitive behavioral treatment, or a combinations of these are treatment alternatives commonly recommended and effective for the treatment of depression in late adulthood.[1] Aside from initiating antidepressant medication or generating a referral to a psychologist, psychiatrist, or other mental health professional for specialized treatment, rehabilitation staff can incorporate multiple strategies in an effort to optimize the performance of the individual with depression. An interdisciplinary approach in which information is shared and treatment plans are collaborative are the ideal structure for such interventions.

As a result of depression or isolation, some older adults may experience a process of increasing inactivity, resulting in prolonged time spent doing sedentary activities or resting in bed during the day. When entering a rehabilitation process, this reduced tolerance to physical activity can make a recovery process more difficult. Inactivity can contribute to frailty, depressed mood, and insomnia. Simple interventions, such as initiating an exercise program, in different modalities has been found to be effective in improving mood symptoms.[12] Rehabilitation providers can also impact mood symptoms through promotion of time spent out of bed, reintegration into leisure activities, and development of a structured schedule based on patients' interests to promote behavioral activation.

Depressed patients will often describe the perception that because of their age they will not improve. Rehabilitation professionals can help the older adult set behavioral goals with short-term targets. In the inpatient setting, daily goals that are agreed to with patients can help promote feelings of achievement in patients experiencing hopelessness and limited motivation. In outpatient clinics, weekly or monthly goals are important to keep patients motivated. Positive reinforcement by a team in which gains are recognized and shared among staff and family members can also help increase participation and motivation toward therapies.

Motivational interviewing is a structured intervention that has been known to help patients set their own goals, identify obstacles that may interfere with that goal, and consider strategies to overcome them. It uses patients' own ideas and knowledge rather than focusing on the health care provider being the expert. Realistic goals that patients identify and can agree to are set. Efforts are made to problem solve around obstacles that may be identified. This process, which can be used by health care professionals from different backgrounds, has been found to be effective in improving chronic pain among the elderly.[13] Seeking training in motivational interviewing can help potentiate a team's ability to achieve change in patients with depression and/or limited interest in working toward change.

Cognitive behavioral therapy helps individuals identify irrational thought patterns that contribute to depressive affect. This form of intervention is provided by a psychotherapist, but other rehabilitation staff can reinforce this effort by assisting patients in challenging cognitions, such as *I can't do anything anymore* or *I'm not useful to anyone*. Evidence to the contrary can be found in patients' daily rehabilitation process, observing interactions with caregivers, and through identification of personal strengths. Helping individuals make these observations rather than informing them of what was noted will be more effective in generating insight and reframing their experience.

Sleep problems can be a symptom of depression or contribute to exacerbation of mood disorders. Interventions, such as sleep hygiene education or cognitive behavioral therapy for insomnia, can be effective interventions for geriatric patients.[14] Sleep hygiene education should be consistently reviewed and reinforced by the rehabilitation team particularly in inpatient settings. Use of medications to treat insomnia can be considered, but with recognition increased risk of side-effect among older adults. Increased risk for falls or mental status changes are some of the possible side effects that have been reported.[15]

Anxiety and the Fear of Falling

Fear and anxiety are appropriate responses to stress or danger and can be useful to help an individual take appropriate precaution. Often anxiety responses become more overwhelming and can paralyze individuals resulting in significant activity limitations. For geriatric patients, anxiety can come from many sources and result in anxiety disorders, including but not limited to posttraumatic stress disorder (PTSD), generalized anxiety disorder, and specific phobias. This section explores anxiety related to fear of falls as a debilitating symptom encountered in older adults undergoing rehabilitation.

Screening for anxiety

Anxiety symptoms are sometimes more difficult for patients to describe given that they manifest themselves in different dimensions. Patients may report feeling anxious but have difficulty putting this into more specific words. The Geriatric Anxiety Scale is a 30-item questionnaire that was designed for and validated with elderly popultations.[16] This scale provides responses in 3 domains: cognitive, somatic, and affective. Results of these domains allow clinicians to identify areas that need to be targeted. Anxiety related to fear of falls can manifest itself in all 3 domains. Patients may experience racing thoughts worrying about the risk and consequence of a fall. Somatic symptoms could include increased respiration rate and bodily tension. Affective response can include irrational fear and restlessness.

Interventions strategies

After geriatric patients experience a fall, fear of falling again can become a debilitating emotion that interferes with the rehabilitation process.[17] This fear can be compounded by experiences in which a geriatric individual who lives alone falls and spends an extended time on the floor unable to receive assistance. Rehabilitation teams often identify patients who become tense, and even rigid, scream, or just avoid the mobility activity altogether because of an anxiety response. These responses are not exclusive to physical or occupational therapy and may also be present when nurses are attempting transfers or bathing. They can also be noted when caregivers are providing assistance. Interventions could include referral to a psychologist for anxiety management strategies, including cognitive behavioral therapy. In some cases, consultation with a psychiatrist for anxiety medication could be indicated as well. Education about anxiety and its effects on the body and mind will be important in normalizing and understanding the anxiety response. Establishing trust is an essential element of overcoming fear of falling. Some patients may erroneously perceive that because a therapist is young, thin, or female, he or she may not be able to help them avoid a fall. Education in this regard with a focus on safety measures, experience, and strategies is essential but probably not sufficient. Patients may also feel pressured to engage in a task they may not be ready for. Exploring what patients are ready to do, providing options, and building on what they are ready to do can make patients feel more comfortable to engage in a particular task. Gradual exposure to more challenging tasks during the course of a therapy session could help desensitize the individual to the feared situations. Use of harnesses during initial phases of training can provide reassurance to fearful patients undergoing mobility training.

Psychologists and other professionals use relaxation strategies to help patients manage anxiety. Diaphragmatic breathing practiced several times before a therapy session and with the addition of visualization of the task can help begin to manage anxiety and cue patients about the need to change the response to the anxiety-provoking situation. Such strategies have been demonstrated to reduce the risk for falling in older adults.[18] In certain occasions, cotreatment in physical therapy or another modality with a psychologist can help patients work through the anxiety and achieve greater gains.

Mindfulness-based interventions have been gaining favor as a tool to manage fear and anxiety. This strategy is accessible to providers from multiple disciplines who seek tools to manage patients in emotional distress. Mindfulness is based on the assumption that thoughts and emotions will be present and if we allow them to pass without judging them or attaching ourselves to them they move on. Mindfulness has been used successfully with geriatric patients to manage chronic pain and anxiety.[19] In a recent study, older adults who were exposed to mindfulness strategies were able to reduce anxiety symptoms and avoidance in a community setting.[20] Use of mindfulness in the context of fear of falling is an area of potential development and research. Exposure through virtual reality has been used for PTSD with some success. Given that falls are traumatic experiences that can result in avoidance and anxiety, this modality is being considered for use in individuals with fear of falling; some positive results have been reported.[21] Recommending a personal alarm system can reduce worry for hospitalized geriatric patients who will be returning to live alone and appropriately fear the possibility of falling.

Clinicians must be aware that some degree of fear is appropriate and may be helpful in preventing falls. Empowering the individual into taking specific steps to reduce falls and avoiding unnecessary risks can give a sense of control over a situation rather than feeling helpless against it.

Adjustment Difficulties in Late Adulthood

Debilitating illnesses and injuries in late adulthood can accelerate loss of function, loss of independence, and changes in roles that can occur naturally during the aging process. Such changes have an impact on perceptions of self-image and self-efficacy. Geriatric patients in rehabilitation often struggle with such concerns compounded by other social circumstances that they may encounter as part of their phase of life.

Changes in roles

Individuals whose sense of identity are strongly related to their professional life, their ability to perform physical tasks, or their role as caregivers/providers often struggle when presented with circumstances in which these roles cannot be performed. Rehabilitation providers are tasked with validating the significance of these changes and the feelings they may bring up while exploring alternatives and problem solving. The ideal goal of rehabilitation would be to recover sufficiently to return to previous levels of function. When this is not possible, using assistive devices/compensatory strategies can allow elderly patients to continue participating in previous activities. Some patients have difficulty with such changes, indicating that *it is just not the same*. Although this can be true, providing opportunities to engage in modified activities or to incorporate assistive devices can serve as behavioral experiments to test the idea that nothing good can come from trying. Behavioral tests are a core element of cognitive behavioral therapy and are important in a rehabilitation process. They serve as opportunities to attempt new approaches, examine results, compare it with preconceived notions, and learn from the experience. Recreational therapy, community-reintegration outings, and living skills therapy are ideal ways of trying out new behaviors and overcoming resistance.

Teaching patients strategies to face present and future difficulties associated with functional problems is an essential component of the rehabilitation process. Problem solving therapy, a psychotherapeutic modality that incorporates this goal, has also been found to have a positive impact on coping and quality of life after stroke.[22] This approach focuses on developing practical strategies to manage challenges of recovery.

Another intervention that can help patients learn new strategies is peer support groups. Such groups present the opportunity to introduce the older adult with individuals who they can identify with. Peers can model positive behaviors and coping strategies, thus, promoting healthier adjustment. Peer support groups have been found to promote social reintegration and knowledge necessary for self-management.[23] Challenges do exist in patients in the creation of such groups among older adults. Difficulty with transportation, comorbid health conditions, and health problems of the caregiver are some of the obstacles that can be observed. Establishing an adequate frequency of meetings based on the group membership characteristics can foster greater commitment and participation. For example, monthly meetings may not be possible for some groups but for others it may be optimal.

Vocational issues and volunteerism

As individuals extend their working careers into old age because of multiple social and economic factors,[24] disabilities resulting from illness or injuries can impact the ability to return to work among geriatric patients. Therefore, a change in function can result in increased stress, economic problems, and changes in role for older adults who are still in the workforce. Health care providers should pay closer attention to this aspect of rehabilitation, because it may be more pressing for patients. Exploring reasonable accommodations and assistive devices can support the employment of the individual in this phase of life. Individuals who may not be able to return to work and perceive themselves as not productive can find in volunteering a way to increase self-esteem and receive the rewards of altruistic behaviors. Volunteerism has been identified as an activity that can promote well-being and positive outcomes in late adulthood.[25] Rehabilitation providers can support these efforts by identifying this activity as a goal for recovery, finding ways of optimizing an individual's ability to overcome challenges imposed by physical limitations, and referring patients to agencies that match organizations with volunteers based on their skills and interests.

Neurocognitive Disorders

A range of cognitive changes are observed in geriatric populations and pose challenges to patients, caregivers, and providers. New classifications in the *DSM-5* include mild neurocognitive disorder, in which there is no significant impact on function or activities of daily living.[26] Major neurocognitive disorder, on the other hand, does suggest impairment in function and activities of daily living. This level of dysfunction is classified through mild, moderate, and severe categories. Cognitive domains in which deficits can be identified include complex attention, executive function, learning and memory, language, perceptual-motor deficits, and social cognition. This section does not focus on causes of these conditions or cognitive rehabilitation, as these are topics for extensive discussion. Rather, how rehabilitation teams can identify and work toward optimizing and achieving rehabilitation goals in the presence of these conditions is explored.

Screening tools

Multiple screening tools have been developed to identify cognitive deficits and contribute to the diagnostic process. Folstein and colleauges'[27] Mini-Mental State Examination (MMSE) is widely used and recognized among health care providers as a tool to screen for cognitive deficits. Even though there are other tests that can provide more information than the MMSE, its widespread use by professionals from across the continuum of care allows for comparisons across time to monitor the course of a disease. The Cognistat[28] is a cognitive screening measure that evaluates 10 different domains and has been found to be valid in geriatric populations. Its usefulness lies in the provision of severity of impairment across the different domains. Also, each domain presents a screen item that if passed the section can be omitted. This function can increase efficiency in administration in settings where there are significant time constraints. The Montreal Cognitive Assessment[29] is a 30-point screening tool that incorporates elements of neuropsychological testing instruments, such as trails, clock drawing, verbal fluency, and verbal learning tests, among others. Scoring does not allow classifying severity but does allow for evaluation for progression of symptoms.

Similarly to other instruments presented in this article, screening tests are not diagnostic. The course of a condition, collateral information, behavioral observations, and functional correlates of deficits observed must also be taken into account. Furthermore, medical and psychological factors that could contribute to presentation must be evaluated. The effect of medications, particularly pain medications and benzodiazepines, should be considered as well. In addition to imaging, laboratory workup including complete blood count, comprehensive metabolic panel (CMP) thyroid function test, test for syphilis (rapid plasma reagin), vitamin B12, folate, human immunodeficiency virus, and toxicology can help identify reversible causes of mental status changes or other causes.[30] A referral for full neuropsychological testing will benefit from completion of these tests before referral in order to facilitate diagnosis.

Intervention Strategies

Individuals with cognitive disorders can experience significant difficulties in rehabilitation as they struggle to learn compensatory strategies, use assistive devices, or perform sequence of steps to achieve a particular activity. Providers and caregivers can experience frustration in their inability to overcome these limitations to achieve rehabilitation goals. One of the most important adaptations in interventions with individuals with cognitive decline is the importance of modifying expectations. Providers must understand the need to repeat information, provide simple instructions, and promote overlearning. Other adaptations can include providing written instructions and using mnemonic strategies to overcome deficits. Literature reviews of research on individuals with dementia recovering from hip fractures have found that individuals with neurocognitive disorder can still benefit from intensive rehabilitation in an inpatient unit.[31] This benefit can be the case if adjustments are made to account for these difficulties and with the support of an interdisciplinary team. Being able to identify specific deficits and relative strengths can help devise interventions that compensate and adjust for patients' difficulties. An individual with attention difficulties may benefit from shorter interventions distributed throughout the day in controlled environments. Others with memory impairment may benefit from longer sessions with more repetition and reinforcement by family members. Referral to a psychologist or neuropsychologist for further input can result in recommendations to guide interventions. Geriatric patients can develop with age changes in vision and hearing. Maximizing an older adult's ability to obtain input from the world will help promote learning in rehabilitation settings. Consults to audiology and a visual examination could help improve performance in the context of rehabilitation.

Exercise has been found to have a positive impact in functional deficits associated with cognitive decline.[32] Promoting an exercise routine in the individual with neurocognitive disorder can also impact mood, energy levels, and social interaction and improve sleep, among other benefits. Rehabilitation efforts with this population should not only strive to achieve rehabilitation goals but also result in patients with dementia incorporating exercise to their daily routine.

Use of compensatory strategies, such as a smartphone and personal digital assistant, have been found to help individuals with dementia reduce functional impairment associated with cognitive decline.[33] The simple interface of many applications can facilitate use of such technologies and become a helpful resource for rehabilitation providers. Keeping a schedule of appointments, writing down reminders or assignments, and playing cognitive stimulating games are just some of the tasks that can be performed with technology that is already part of patients' lives.

Incorporating caregivers in the rehab process of elderly patients with neurocognitive disorder can help reinforce the areas or skills that are being addressed. It can also help empower the caregivers to familiarize themselves with the tasks that they will need to assume and help reduce anxiety related to the return home after hospitalization.

Caregiver Support

Caring for an individual with a neurocognitive disorder, stroke, and other debilitating conditions can have profound impact on individuals, who may experience burnout, depression, and declining health. Caregivers who are well informed and empowered can provide more efficient care for a longer period of time. Assessment tools have been developed to screen for caregiver burden. These tools can help identify caregivers who are at risk of developing physical and mental health problems associated with their new role. The Zarit Burden Interview[34] explores, through 22 items, perception of burden among caregivers. Such a scale can help initiate a conversation with a caregiver about the importance of self-care and, when possible, seeking support from other family members. Promoting participation in support groups, educational activities, and, when necessary, recommending mental health treatment are strategies that have been deemed beneficial in helping prevent burnout.[35]

Perceptions on Aging and Resilience

Some individuals may have a predefined perception about aging that shapes the way this stage of life evolves. Studies have reported that individuals who have negative perceptions of aging are more likely to develop frailty and cognitive impairment.[36] The mechanism that mediates these processes may be complex. However, promoting healthy perspectives on aging and the changes that are to be expected is deemed to be important and beneficial. Health care providers must also be aware of their own predetermined notions of late adulthood, because these may reinforce negative perceptions of aging that patients may already have.

Resilience, on the other hand, involves the ability to withstand significant challenges through the use of positive coping mechanisms and a perspective that personal growth can be accomplished at any age.[37] One way resilience can be promoted is through the use of reminiscence or remembering/retelling the past with the purpose of seeing what elements of patients' identities do not change and finding meaning in the experiences that are encountered. Providers can promote resilience through helping patients reframe their current experiences, reinforce personal strengths, and explore how they have coped with similar challenges in the past.

SUMMARY

This article reviews a selection of the many psychosocial issues encountered in the rehabilitation of individuals in geriatric populations. Increasing awareness and skills in the management of these factors can help rehabilitation providers overcome barriers and promote functional gains. Optimizing wellness in this population rests in a provider's or teams' ability to perform a comprehensive assessment that can identify psychosocial factors. A comprehensive geriatric assessment by nonspecialists has been promoted by Welsh and colleagues[38] as a way to foster adequate management and optimization of older adults. In this model, in addition to functional problems, mood, fears, cognition, and social circumstances are considered. Another such effort targets a comprehensive geriatric assessment in the context of neurocognitive disorder. The Dementia Dashboard[39] is an approach that seeks to reduce risks through comprehensive evaluation and management of risk factors, such as depression, caregiver distress, risk of falls, medication management/errors, driving, and transportation, among others. The physical medicine and rehabilitation physician and other rehabilitation providers are encouraged to examine and consider the full complexity of geriatric patients in order to maximize gains and foster wellness.

REFERENCES

1. Edelstein B, Bamonti P, Gregg J, et al. Depression in later life. In: Lichtenberg P, Mast B, editors. APA handbook of clinical geropsychology. Assessment, treatment, and issues of later life. vol. 2. Washington, DC: American Psychological Association; 2015. p. 3–48.
2. Hörnsten C, Lövheim H, Nordström P, et al. The prevalence of stroke and depression and factors associated with depression in elderly people with and without stroke. BMC Geriatr 2016;16(1):174.

3. Buijck B, Zuidema S, Spruit-van Eijk M, et al. Determinants of geriatric patients' quality of life after stroke rehabilitation. Aging Ment Health 2014;18(8):980–5.
4. Reyes R, Leahey E, Leahey E. Elderly patients with lower extremity amputations: three-year study in a rehabilitation setting. Arch Phys Med Rehabil 1977;58(3): 116–23.
5. Vasiliadis H, Dionne P, Préville M, et al. The excess healthcare costs associated with depression and anxiety in elderly living in the community. Am J Geriatr Psychiatry 2013;21(6):536–48.
6. Lin E, Katon W, Unützer J, et al. Effect of improving depression care on pain and functional outcomes among older adults with arthritis: a randomized controlled trial. JAMA 2003;290(18):2428–9.
7. Gallo J, Rabins P. Depression without sadness: alternative presentations of depression in late life. Am Fam Physician 1999;60(3):820–6.
8. Pocklington C, Gilbody S, Manea L, et al. The diagnostic accuracy of brief versions of the geriatric depression scale: a systematic review and meta-analysis. Int J Geriatr Psychiatry 2016;31(8):837–57.
9. Conradsson M, Rosendahl E, Littbrand H, et al. Usefulness of the geriatric depression scale 15-item version among very old people with and without cognitive impairment. Aging Ment Health 2013;17(5):638–45.
10. Costa M, Diniz M, Diniz B, et al. Accuracy of three depression screening scales to diagnose major depressive episodes in older adults without neurocognitive disorders. Rev Bras Psiquiatr 2016;38(2):154–6.
11. Sackley C, Hoppitt T, Cardoso K. An investigation into the utility of the stroke aphasic depression questionnaire (SADQ) in care home settings. Clin Rehabil 2006;20(7):598–602.
12. Villada F, Vélez E, Baena L. Ejercicio físico y depresión en adultos mayores: Una revisión sistemática. = Physical exercise and depression in the elderly: a systematic review. Rev Colomb Psiquiatr 2013;42(2):198–211 [Article in Spanish].
13. Tse M, Vong S, Tang S. Motivational interviewing and exercise programme for community-dwelling older persons with chronic pain: a randomized controlled study. J Clin Nurs 2013;22(13–14):1843–56.
14. Medina-Chávez J, Fuentes-Alexandro S, Sánchez-Narváez F, et al. Clinical practice guideline. Diagnosis and treatment of insomnia in the elderly. Rev Med Inst Mex Seguro Soc 2014;52(1):108–19 [Article in Spanish].
15. Davies E, O'Mahony M. Adverse drug reactions in special populations - the elderly. Br J Clin Pharmacol 2015;80(4):796–807.
16. Mueller A, Segal D, Coolidge F, et al. Geriatric anxiety scale: item response theory analysis, differential item functioning, and creation of a ten-item short form (GAS-10). Int Psychogeriatr 2015;27(7):1099–111.
17. Visschedijk J, Caljouw M, Bakkers E, et al. Longitudinal follow-up study on fear of falling during and after rehabilitation in skilled nursing facilities. BMC Geriatr 2015;15:161.
18. Kim B, Newton R, Sachs M, et al. Effect of guided relaxation and imagery on falls self-efficacy: a randomized controlled trial. J Am Geriatr Soc 2012;60(6):1109–14.
19. Morone N, Greco C, Weiner D, et al. A mind-body program for older adults with chronic low back pain: a randomized clinical trial. JAMA Intern Med 2016;176(3): 329–37.
20. Perez-Blasco J, Sales A, Meléndez J, et al. The effects of mindfulness and self-compassion on improving the capacity to adapt to stress situations in elderly people living in the community. Clin Gerontol 2016;39(2):90–103.

21. Marivan K, Boully C, Bloch F, et al. Rehabilitation of the psychomotor consequences of falling in an elderly population: a pilot study to evaluate feasibility and tolerability of virtual reality training. Technol Health Care 2016; 24(2):169–75.

22. Visser M, Heijenbrok-Kal M, Van't Spijker A, et al. Problem-solving therapy during outpatient stroke rehabilitation improves coping and health-related quality of life: randomized controlled trial. Stroke 2016;47(1):135–42.

23. Weltermann B, Homann J, Ringelstein E, et al. Stroke knowledge among stroke support group members. Stroke 2000;31(6):1230–3.

24. Sterns H, McQuown C. Retirement redefined. In: Lichtenberg P, Mast B, editors. APA handbook of clinical geropsychology, assessment, treatment, and issues of later life, vol. 2. Washington, DC: American Psychological Association; 2015. p. 601–16.

25. Kahana E, Bhatta T, Lovegreen L, et al. Altruism, helping, and volunteering: pathways to well-being in late life. J Aging Health 2013;25(1):159–87.

26. American Psychiatric Association. Diagnostic and statistical manual of mental disorder. 5th edition. Washington, DC: American Psychiatric Association; 2013.

27. Folstein MF, Folstein SE, McHugh PR. Mini-Mental State: a practical method for grading the cognitive state of patients for the clinician. J Psychiatr Res 1975; 12(3):189–98.

28. Mueller J, Kiernan R, Langston JW. Cognistat (Neurobehavioral cognitive status examination). Fairfax (NC): Neurobehavioral Group; 2001.

29. Nasreddine ZS, Phillips NA, Bédirian V, et al. The Montreal Cognitive Assessment, MoCA: a brief screening tool for mild cognitive impairment. J Am Geriatr Soc 2005;53(4):695–9.

30. Thakur ME, Doraiswamy PM. Use of the laboratory in the diagnostic workup of older adults. In: Blazer DG, Steffent DC, editors. Essentials Geriatric Psychiatry. Washington DC: American Psychiatric Publishing; 2012. p. 63–74.

31. Resnick B, Beaupre L, Magaziner J, et al. Rehabilitation interventions for older individuals with cognitive impairment post-hip fracture: a systematic review. J Am Med Dir Assoc 2016;17(3):200–5.

32. Laver K, Dyer S, Whitehead C, et al. Interventions to delay functional decline in people with dementia: a systematic review of systematic reviews. BMJ Open 2016;6(4):e010767.

33. Svoboda E, Richards B, Yao C, et al. Long-term maintenance of smartphone and PDA use in individuals with moderate to severe memory impairment. Neuropsychol Rehabil 2015;25(3):353–73.

34. Zarit SH, Reever KE, Bach-Peterson J. Relatives of the impaired elderly: correlations of feelings of burden. Gerontologist 1980;20(6):649–55.

35. Zarit S, Heid A. Assessment and treatment of family caregivers. In: Lichtenberg P, Mast B, editors. APA handbook of clinical geropsychology. Assessment, treatment, and issues of later life, vol. 2. Washington, DC: American Psychological Association; 2015. p. 521–51.

36. Robertson D, Kenny R. Negative perceptions of aging modify the association between frailty and cognitive function in older adults. Pers Individ Dif 2016; 100(1):120–5. Available at: E-Journals, Ipswich, MA. Available at: http://www.sciencedirect.com/science/article/pii/S019188691530091X. Accessed March 2, 2017.

37. Aldwin C, Igarashi H. Successful, optimal, and resilient aging: a psychosocial perspective. In: Lichtenberg P, Mast B, editors. APA handbook of clinical

geropsychology. History and status of the field and perspectives on aging, vol. 1. Washington, DC: American Psychological Association; 2015. p. 331–59.

38. Welsh T, Gordon A, Gladman J. Comprehensive geriatric assessment–a guide for the non-specialist. Int J Clin Pract 2014;68(3):290–3.

39. Dalsania P. Dementia dashboard a proactive risk reduction management guideline. Top Geriatr Rehabil 2006;22(3):228–42.

Physiologic Changes of the Musculoskeletal System with Aging: A Brief Review

Walter R. Frontera, MD, PhD[a,b,*]

KEYWORDS

- Older adults • Skeletal muscle • Weakness • Sarcopenia

KEY POINTS

- The number and percentage of people in older age groups is increasing significantly in most countries of the world resulting in important socioeconomic and health challenges.
- Many components of the musculoskeletal system, including skeletal muscle, tendons, ligaments, bone, and articular cartilage, show significant losses of structural and functional properties.
- Age-associated changes in musculoskeletal tissues compromised an individual's capacity to perform many activities of daily living as well as more demanding tasks.
- Many of the age-associated changes seen in the musculoskeletal system can be partially modified with an active lifestyle and appropriate exercise training.

INTRODUCTION

The World Health Organization has recognized the aging of the population in many countries around the world as one of the most significant challenges of the twenty-first century.[1] In several countries in Asia and Europe, the average life expectancy has already exceeded 80 years, particularly among women. In fact, the fastest growing age group in the United States is the oldest-old (>85 years) group. It has been estimated that by the year 2025, the number of people older than 60 years in the planet will exceed 1 billion and 2 billion by the year 2050.[1,2] Although there are significant differences between countries associated with sociopolitical conditions and the level of income, the increase in life expectancy and in the number of people in this age group has been documented in low-, middle-, and high-income countries.[3]

Disclosure: The author has nothing to disclose.
[a] Departments of Physical Medicine, Rehabilitation, and Sports Medicine, School of Medicine, University of Puerto Rico, PO Box 365067, San Juan, PR 00936-5067, USA; [b] Department of Physiology, School of Medicine, University of Puerto Rico, PO Box 365067, San Juan, PR 00936-5067, USA
* Departments of Physical Medicine, Rehabilitation, and Sports Medicine, School of Medicine, University of Puerto Rico, PO Box 365067, San Juan, PR 00936-5067.
E-mail address: walter.frontera@upr.edu

It should not come as a surprise that these changes in the age-group composition of the population have significant social, economic, political, and health implications.[4] Thus, understanding age-related changes in human physiology and their consequences is of significant interest and relevance and has been identified as a research priority by the US National Institutes of Health.[5]

The main challenge associated with advanced adult age is the relationship between significant alterations in many physiologic functions, the development of multiple impairments, the decline in overall functional capacity, the associated morbidity and mortality, and the resulting loss of independence that most older adults fear more than death. For example, because maximal physiologic capacities are greatly diminished with age, the ability to perform physical tasks at the same absolute level of energy expenditure or muscular force becomes limited. In other words, activities such as rising from a chair or crossing a city street intersection that usually represent submaximal demands can become, in old age, maximal or impossible efforts (**Fig. 1**). It should also be noted that physical or architectural obstacles may contribute to this problem by making the environment less friendly.

Some of the most important contributors to the functional loss leading to impairment and disability are the multiple changes in structure and function of the musculoskeletal system. Left unchecked, life-threatening complications, such as falls and bone fractures associated with muscle weakness, can occur. In fact, mortality after a fall resulting in a fracture is higher in those with a lower level of muscle strength before the fall. The biological changes resulting from aging contribute to a decline in skeletal muscle strength and mass, alterations in muscle contractile properties, impaired motor performance, a reduction in bone mass and strength, a decrease in flexibility and joint range of motion, and the loss of the capacity of soft tissues to sustain and recover from injury. It is interesting that the qualitative nature of these changes is very similar to those experienced during the inactivity that follows injury or hospitalization underlining the contribution of a sedentary life, inactivity, and immobilization to the age-associated loss of function and independence.

MUSCLE STRENGTH

Skeletal muscle strength is one of the fundamental physiologic capacities that contribute to functional capacity. Muscle strength alone is a strong predictor of severe mobility limitation, slow gait speed, increased fall risk, risk of hospitalization, and high mortality rate. For example, older adults with poor muscle strength have a 2.6-fold

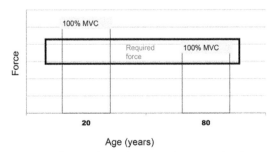

Fig. 1. Force required to rise from a chair relative to the strength of a person. At 20 years of age, the maximal voluntary contraction (MVC) is much higher than the force required to perform a simple task, such as rising from a chair. Because of the reduction in muscle strength with aging, the same task may represent a maximal effort in an 80-year-old person.

greater risk of severe mobility limitation, a 4.3-fold greater risk for slow gait speed, and a 2.1-fold greater risk of mortality compared with older adults with high muscle strength.[6]

Aging is associated with a significant reduction in muscle strength, defined as the capacity to generate maximal force at a specified velocity (zero in the case of isometric/static muscle actions). Cross-sectional studies have shown that both older men and women have lower strength in multiple upper and lower limb muscle groups when compared with their younger counterparts. Furthermore, longitudinal studies have shown that this reduction in muscle strength is approximately 1.0% to 1.5% per year[7] and it is more noticeable in the lower limbs (knee extensors and flexors) of men and women and almost nonexistent in the upper limbs in women. Equally relevant, and perhaps more significant from a functional point of view, is the reduction in muscle power or the product of force times velocity.[8] This reduction has been estimated to be approximately 2.9% per year and is very important because the successful performance of many activities of daily living depends more on the generation of a certain level of force quickly than in maximal levels of force that are almost never required during daily life.

One factor that may contribute to a decline in muscle strength and power is the reduction in the ability to activate motor units. This point is particularly true in healthy older humans who are not mobility impaired.[8] Both central and peripheral factors may contribute to this reduction in neuromuscular activation, including a decline in central nervous system drive, changes at the level of the spinal cord, and alterations of the peripheral nerve and neuromuscular junction. On the other hand, in the case of mobility-impaired patients, the loss of muscle power is due to a combination of deficits in muscle strength and contraction velocity.

MUSCLE SIZE

Skeletal muscle comprises approximately 40% of the human body weight and contains between 50% and 70% of all proteins in the human body. Therefore, muscle atrophy is an important determinant of muscle dysfunction in elderly. The correlation between muscle strength and muscle size is positive but not perfect, and the age-associated reduction in strength is only partially due to the loss of muscle mass.

This loss of muscle mass together with changes in function (walking speed) and strength is known as sarcopenia.[9] It has been known for several years that both a decline in the number of muscle fibers (mainly those expressing type II myosin heavy chain isoform) and a reduction in muscle fiber size contribute to muscle atrophy in older men and women.[10] Sarcopenia affects muscles of both upper and lower limbs as well as the paraspinal muscle group.[11] It must be noted that these changes in muscle mass seen on imaging studies are accompanied by increases in fat and changes in muscle density that correlate well with changes in muscle function.

MUSCLE QUALITY AND ALTERATIONS IN SINGLE MUSCLE FIBERS

The concept of muscle quality has been developed to indicate alterations in muscle function that are independent of changes in muscle mass or size (cross-sectional area). At the macroscopic level, these changes are reflected in reductions in muscle density as measured with MRI studies and increases in intermuscular fat.[11] At the single fiber level, older people have lower specific force or force adjusted for differences in muscle fiber size (a physiologic index of muscle quality).[12] It is interesting that longitudinal studies show that surviving fibers may maintain normal strength and shortening velocity in an attempt to compensate for the fibers that have been lost as a result of the aging process.[13]

DETERMINANTS OF FORCE, POWER, MOVEMENT, AND FUNCTION

There are 4 general domains that contribute to the capacity of skeletal muscle to generate force, power, and movement.[14] These 4 domains are structure and architecture, fiber type distribution, excitation-contraction coupling, and energy release. There is very good scientific evidence in support of age-related alterations in all 4 domains. (**Table 1**) For example, as mentioned earlier, the number of muscle fibers is reduced with age, particularly fibers expressing type II myosin heavy chain isoform. This loss of muscle fibers is accompanied by a reduction in average muscle fiber cross-sectional area of both type I and II fibers. Skeletal muscle may not be able to compensate for this loss because regeneration of muscle fibers is limited because of a reduction in the number of satellite cells, particularly those associated with type II fibers. Furthermore, activation of existing satellite cells is also impaired. As a consequence of this, fiber type distribution is altered with a small increase in the percent of type I fibers, a significant reduction in type II fibers, and an increase in the number of hybrid fibers expressing more than one myosin heavy chain at the same time. The functional significance of these hybrid fibers is unknown, but some investigators considered them to be immature fibers or fibers in transition. Further, significant alterations and fragmentation in the triad, including the t-tubule and sarcoplasmic reticulum system, result in impaired calcium release and uncoupling of the excitation-contraction processes. Finally, some studies, but not all, demonstrate significant impairment of oxidative pathways, including a reduction in mitochondrial volume and capacity. Various combinations of the changes described earlier result in an impaired capacity to perform a spectrum of activities typical of daily life that have different power demands.

The mechanical process at the molecular level that underlies muscle weakness is a dysfunctional formation and interaction of actin-myosin cross-bridges. The number of cross-bridges in the strong-binding state is lower in aged muscle resulting in muscle weakness. Similarly, the dissociation of actin and myosin that determines the shortening velocity of the muscle fiber is impaired. One of the explanations for these changes is the presence of posttranslational chemical alterations of motor proteins, such as myosin including glycation and oxidation. In other words, biochemical alterations known to occur with aging can explain some of the functional alterations in muscle force and power production.[15]

Table 1
Summary of age-related changes in skeletal muscle

Muscle strength	Lower
Muscle mass	Lower
Muscle quality	Increase in fat and connective tissue
Fiber number	Lower (particularly type II)
Fiber type distribution	Increase type I and reduced type II
Fiber specific force	Lower
Excitation-contraction coupling	Impaired (uncoupling and fragmentation of cellular elements)
Energy release	Reduced oxidative capacity
Muscle proteins (myosin)	Altered because of biochemical changes
Satellite cells	Decline in those associated with type II fibers

TENDONS

Tendons are important anatomic structures because they transmit the force developed by muscle cells to bones, making movement possible. The fundamental biochemical component of tendon is type I collagen organized in fibrils that represent the force-transmitting unit of the tendon. These fibrils are stabilized and strengthened by cross-links between collagen molecules and embedded in extracellular matrix composed of cells (fibroblasts) and proteoglycans. Tendons respond to mechanical loading and unloading and are at risk of injury during activities, such as daily household activities, work-related activities, exercise training, and sports participation.

The effect of aging on tendon structure and function has been recently reviewed.[16,17] Tendon tissue injuries seem to be more frequent with aging, including the tendons of the rotator cuff, the patellar tendon, and the Achilles tendon. It has been suggested that genetic factors may contribute to tendinopathy in older patients with rotator cuff disease.[18] When compared with immature tissue, the most important effects of aging on tendons include a reduction in cell density, a decline in matrix turnover, an increase in cross-links particularly in nonenzymatic cross-links called advanced glycation end products, a mild reduction in fibril diameter, and a reduction in the elastic modulus. The importance of glycation is that it increases the distance between collagen molecules and reduces water content. These alterations change the mechanical properties of the tissue resulting in an increased susceptibility to injury. Finally, short-term immobilization (2 weeks) of human elderly tendon reduces collagen protein synthesis, although no significant change in mechanical properties was noted.[19] It has been suggested that the effects of aging and exercise on tendons are mediated via changes on tendon stem/progenitor cells. In other words, aging impairs proliferation of stem cells and reduces its ability to regenerate, whereas exercise increases proliferation of stem cells.[20]

LIGAMENTS

Ligaments provide important joint support and stability. From biochemical and biomechanical points of view, the changes in ligaments seen with aging are similar to those described earlier for tendons.[16,21] These changes include decreases in collagen synthesis and concentration, elastic modulus (an indication of accumulated damage and risk for further damage), and ultimate force. Similarly, there is an increase in failure strain. Further, the expression of some proteoglycans that serve as lubricants on the surface of the ligament and between collagen fiber bundles is increased. It has been suggested that these changes taken together explain the higher incidence of ligamentous injuries in older people.[22]

BONE

A well-known change in bone health with advanced adult age is a reduction in bone mineral content and density. In the United States, recent data from the National Health and Nutrition Examination Survey show that the prevalence of osteoporosis in adult (aged 50+ years) women was 9.8% (femur), 11.6% (lumbar spine), and 16.5% (either femur neck or lumbar spine) depending on the anatomic area studied.[23] In general, this study suggests a higher prevalence in osteoporosis compared with 2007 to 2008. Further, the prevalence of low bone mass ranged from 36% to 53%, also in women. Both conditions were found in men, but the prevalence was significantly higher in women. In addition, non-Hispanic blacks showed a lower prevalence of osteoporosis and low bone mass.

The presence of osteoporosis and/or low bone mass contributes to the high risk for fractures in the elderly because it increases bone fragility. This risk is complicated by the fact that mechanical loading in the form of physical activity is reduced in older people.[24] It has been proposed that dynamic mechanical loading, and not only weight-bearing activities, is required to strengthen bone architecture. There is good scientific evidence from clinical trials of the benefits of exercise training on bone mineral density in older adults.[25]

The various components of the musculoskeletal system interact with each other and influence their individual response to the aging process. Changes in both muscle and bone tissues can result in significant impairment and disability. Thus, it is important to note that components of sarcopenia (reduced muscle strength, mass, and performance) are significantly associated with osteoporosis.[26]

ARTICULAR CARTILAGE

The effects of aging on articular cartilage and related tissues has been recently reviewed.[27] Aging is associated with a higher prevalence of chondrocytes that have lost their ability to divide (diminished mitotic activity). The loss of chondrocytes is facilitated by trauma and excessive mechanical loading and may be mediated by increased oxidative stress associated with loading. In addition, older chondrocytes have reduced ability to synthesize components of the extracellular matrix, such as collagen and ground substance.

Stiffness of the collagen network in many tissues, including articular cartilage, increases with age because of an increase in cross-links by advanced glycation end products. The functional consequence of these changes is a reduction in the capacity for deformation that may lead to injury. Finally, the synthesis of proteoglycans, an important component of the ground substance, is decreased with advanced adult age.

It is interesting to note that lack of mechanical stimulation, typical of bed rest and immobilization prevalent in old age, results in thinner and softer articular cartilage. Some studies have suggested that exercise training has the opposite effect.

SUMMARY

The musculoskeletal system undergoes significant changes with advanced adult age. The structural and functional properties of all the tissue elements of the system change reducing their capacity to enhance mobility and withstand injury. More research is needed to understand the mechanisms underlying these losses and the potential of physical activity and exercise to preserve more normal tissue characteristics.

REFERENCES

1. World Health Organization. World report on ageing and health. Geneva (Switzerland); 2015.
2. Available at: www.who.org. Accessed March 20, 2017.
3. Stucki G, Bickenbach J, Gutenbrunner C, et al. Rehabilitation: the health strategy of the 21st century. J Rehabil Med 2017. http://dx.doi.org/10.2340/16501977-2200.
4. Harper S. Economic and social implications of aging societies. Science 2014; 346:587–91.
5. Frontera WR, Bean JF, Damiano D, et al. Rehabilitation research at the National Institutes of Health: moving the field forward (executive summary). Am J Phys Med Rehabil 2017;96:211–20.

6. Manini TM. Development of physical disability in older adults. Curr Aging Sci 2011;4:184–91.
7. Frontera WR, Hughes VA, Fielding RA, et al. Aging of skeletal muscle: a 12-yr longitudinal study. J Appl Physiol (1985) 2000;88:1321–6.
8. Reid KF, Pasha E, Doros G, et al. Longitudinal decline of lower extremity muscle power in healthy and mobility-limited older adults: influence of muscle mass, strength, composition, neuromuscular activation and single fiber contractile properties. Eur J Appl Physiol 2014;114:29–39.
9. Cruz-Jentoft AJ, Baeyens JP, Bauer JM, et al. Sarcopenia: European consensus on definition and diagnosis. Age Ageing 2010;39:412–23.
10. Lexell J, Taylor CC, Sjostrom M. What is the cause of the ageing atrophy? Total number, size, and proportion of different fiber types studied in whole vastus lateralis muscle from15- to 83-year-old men. J Neurol Sci 1988;84:275–94.
11. Dahlqvist JR, Vissing CR, Hermann G, et al. Fat replacement of paraspinal muscles with aging in healthy adults. Med Sci Sports Exerc 2017;49:595–601.
12. Frontera WR, Krivickas L, Suh D, et al. Skeletal muscle fiber quality in older men and women. Am J Physiol Cell Physiol 2000;279:C611–8.
13. Frontera WR, Reid KF, Phillips EM, et al. Muscle fiber size and function in elderly humans: a longitudinal study. J Appl Physiol 2008;105:637–42.
14. Frontera WR, Ochala J. Skeletal muscle: a brief review of structure and function. Calcif Tissue Int 2014;96:183–95.
15. Li M, Ogilvie H, Ochala J, et al. Aberrant post-translational modifications compromise human myosin motor function in old age. Aging Cell 2015;14:228–35.
16. McCarthy MM, Hannafin JA. The mature athlete: aging tendon and ligament. Sports Health 2014;6:41–8.
17. Svensson RB, Heinemeier KM, Couppé C, et al. Effect of aging and exercise on the tendon. J Appl Physiol 2016;121:1353–62.
18. Dabija DI, Gao C, Edwards TL, et al. Genetic and familial predisposition to rotator cuff disease: a systematic review. J Shoulder Elbow Surg 2017;26(6):1103–12.
19. Dideriksen K, Boesen AP, Reitelseder S, et al. Tendon collagen synthesis declines with immobilization in elderly humans: no effect of anti-inflammatory medication. J Appl Physiol 2017;122:273–82.
20. Zhang J, Wang JHC. Moderate exercise mitigates the detrimental effects of aging on tendon stem cells. PLoS One 2015;10(6):e0130454.
21. Thornton GM, Lemmex DB, Ono Y, et al. Aging affects mechanical properties and lubricin/PRG4 gene expression in normal ligaments. J Biomech 2015;48:3306–11.
22. Haapasalo H, Parkkari J, Kannus P, et al. Knee injuries in leisure-time physical activities: a prospective one-year follow-up of a Finnish population cohort. Int J Sports Med 2007;28:72–7.
23. Looker AC, Sarafrazi Isfahani N, Fan B, et al. Trends in osteoporosis and low bone mass in older US adults, 2005-2006 through 2013-2014. Osteoporos Int 2017;28(6):1979–88.
24. Sugiyama T, Oda H. Osteoporosis therapy: bone modeling during growth and aging. Front Endocrinol (Lausanne) 2017;8:46.
25. Marques EA, Mota J, Carvalho J. Exercise effects on bone mineral density in older adults: a meta-analysis of randomized controlled trials. Age 2012;34:1493–515.
26. Sjöblom S, Suuronen J, Rikkonen T, et al. Relationship between postmenopausal osteoporosis and the components of clinical sarcopenia. Maturitas 2013;75:175–80.
27. Jørgensen AE, Kjær M, Heinemeir KM. The effect of aging and mechanical loading on the metabolism of articular cartilage. J Rheumatol 2017;44(4):410–7.

Normal Changes in Gait and Mobility Problems in the Elderly

Maricarmen Cruz-Jimenez, MD[a,b,*]

KEYWORDS

• Elderly • Gait • Mobility • Lower extremity

KEY POINTS

- Gait and mobility are altered with aging, and these changes are a combination of alterations in the gait pattern and in the function of organs.
- Changes in gait are associated with functional decline, less independence, and impaired quality of life.
- Reduced walking speed is the most consistent age-related change, but there are other contributors to an altered gait: impaired balance and stability, lower extremity strength, and the fear of falling.

BACKGROUND

There are normal physiologic changes that occur as the body ages. These changes affect the body, organs, and systems, and their functional decline may alter general function and abilities that eventually impair independence and quality of life.[1] As people age, gait and mobility are altered too as posture and the typical movement patterns involved in walking change. However, these changes are not limited by alterations in movement patterns alone, but by the decline in function of other organs whose role contributes to this complex physiologic activity. Gait speed is a specific variable used to study the declining function of mobility. This correlation between gait speed and other organs is such that the deterioration of gait speed has been related to the risk of mortality, the volume of medical care, hospitalizations, onset of activities of daily living (ADL) disability, and nursing home placement.[2] As rehabilitators, it is essential for clinicians to understand that maintaining ambulation is not limited to functional independence but is related to general health and wellness, and that their role should include early identification of changing patterns that lead to preventive interventions.

Disclosure: The author has nothing to disclose.
[a] Physical Medicine and Rehabilitation, VA Caribbean Healthcare System, San Juan, PR, USA;
[b] Physical Medicine and Rehabilitation, University of Puerto Rico, San Juan, PR, USA
* Physical Medicine and Rehabilitation, VA Caribbean Healthcare System, San Juan, PR.
E-mail address: Maricarmen.Cruz-Jimenez@va.gov

Phys Med Rehabil Clin N Am 28 (2017) 713–725
http://dx.doi.org/10.1016/j.pmr.2017.06.005
1047-9651/17/Published by Elsevier Inc.

HUMAN WALKING

Gait and mobility are not the same thing. Human gait refers to a walking style, to the locomotion achieved by using the human limbs. It is a bipedal activity that displaces the center of gravity forward. Mobility is the ability to displace in the environment with ease, and without restriction. It does not imply necessarily using the limbs to move the body from one place to another. Mobility disability in adults is an important factor for loss of independence.

There are two components that are fundamental to the ability to walk: equilibrium and locomotion. Based on Nutt and colleagues,[3] equilibrium is the capacity to assume an upright posture and maintain balance. Locomotion is the ability to initiate and maintain rhythmic steps.

In order to maintain an upright posture, the erect spine rests on the sacral base, and conforms its natural curves to the center of gravity. To attain stability, the spine balances both static and dynamic functions, including weight bearing and balance, and it accomplishes the task by using structures like the anterior vertebrae, both anterior and posterior longitudinal ligaments, facets, and spinal muscles. Seeking energy conservation, the center of gravity is kept within the boundary created by the feet in its base of support, and the static balanced spine posture takes advantage of ground reaction forces to minimize muscle activation. These forces strategically cross the naturally conformed spine curves and the lower extremity joints, allowing balanced and static control (**Fig. 1**). When the spine moves off the balanced posture, there is three-dimensional motion of the spine, causing simultaneous coupling of flexion, lateral flexion, and rotation of the muscles of the spine.[4] Patla and colleagues[5] reported that simple movements in the balanced posture, like arm elevation, deviate the center of mass (COM) away from its center, and proportionately relative to the length of the base of support. There is neurologic control that enhances the precision of this COM displacement and how the body compensates to maintain dynamic

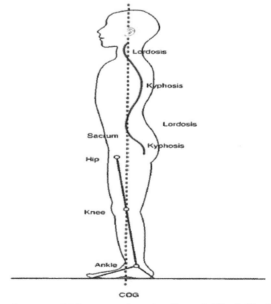

Fig. 1. The balanced posture. COG, center of gravity. (*From* Cailliet R. The illustrated guide to functional anatomy of the musculoskeletal system. 2004 American Medical; with permission.)

balance. Once the COM moves, reaction forces activate and act on other body joints, particularly those in the lower extremity. Active control of muscles at the hip, knee, and ankle is then required to prevent the body from collapsing. The specifics of how joint control is achieved can be understood by studying the gait cycle.

Walking is basic in human motion and can be studied by assessing the gait cycle. This cycle is a combination of steps and swings by the legs, and is described from the moment one foot strikes the ground until that same foot returns to the ground (**Fig. 2**). As the cycle repeats, the body displaces in space for a specific distance. That segment or distance covered from one foot strike to striking the ground again is called stride (**Fig. 3**). The distance covered by each foot is called step, and is symmetric in length for both sides. The frequency of stepping is called cadence, and it is described as the number of steps per minute. To calculate the walking speed, the cadence is multiplied by the step length.[6]

Normal gait is a complex activity that involves a series of rhythmic and alternating movements of the trunk and limbs, and that seeks to perform to the lowest energy cost. To achieve an energy-efficient ambulation, there is a synchronized pattern of movements at the foot, ankle, knee, hip, and pelvis. The lower extremity muscles involved take advantage of ground reaction forces, momentum, and posture to minimize active contractions that consume energy, and this consequently allows a smooth flow of motion while providing stability. These principles were established by the studies of Saunders and colleagues,[7] who described the six determinants for the gait cycle, which have become key to understanding normal locomotion and why deviations from normal affect the efficiency of natural walking. The six determinants operate independently of each other, but simultaneously to produce the minimal displacement of the center of gravity (COG). This COG is considered to be localized at about 55% of the height of the individual, and just in front of the second sacral vertebrae. The six determinants are pelvis rotation, pelvic tilt, knee flexion in stance phase, foot mechanism, knee mechanism, and lateral displacement of the pelvis (**Table 1**). Kinematic studies explain the angular relationship of the lower extremity segments as they move, whereas kinetic studies explain the forces that produce and/or inhibit motion. It is through the combination of joint motion and the contraction and inhibition of muscles that a stable ambulation pattern is attained at the lowest energy cost.

During ambulation, people use an optimal walking speed, which is a self-selected gait speed at which they are comfortable. At this rate, the body is efficient in its energy consumption. Increasing the walking speed leads to increasing the muscle energy

The Gait Cycle

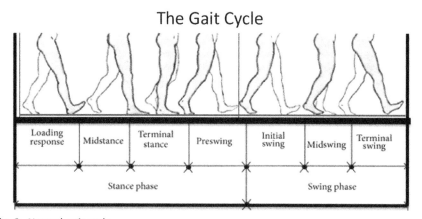

Fig. 2. Normal gait cycle.

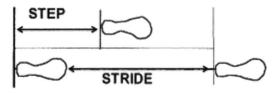

Fig. 3. Stride and step.

requirements and the total basal body metabolism, which copes with the increased activity demand. When this occurs, other body systems are required to adapt their basal activity to cope with the physiologic request, as seen, for example, in the heart and the respiratory systems when they increase the pulse rate and respiratory frequency.

As people learn to walk, there are central and peripheral neuroadaptations that lead to a mature walking pattern. It takes about 12 months for a human to learn to walk, and about 10 years to master the gait pattern. Sutherland and colleagues[8] describe that gait is considered mature when the following five determinants are observed: duration of the single limb stance, walking velocity, cadence, step length, and the ratio of pelvic span to angle spread. Other characteristics of mature gait include reciprocating arm swing and the reduction of unnecessary muscle activation. Once walking is mastered, it becomes an automatic task that requires minimal conscious effort.

GAIT DEVIATIONS WITH AGING
Gait Parameters

The characteristic patterns of gait and mobility of an old adult include postural and balance changes as psychomotor skills decline. The prevalence of gait disorders among elders more than 70 years of age is estimated to be 35%.[9] Although this is considered significant, 85% of 60-year-olds and 20% of people more than 85 years old can still walk normally.[10] When referring to age-related changes, some investigators use the term senile gait disorders to describe patterns in the elderly that include a slow pace, broad base, shuffling, and cautious walking. Evidence has shown that gait patterns like this are not idiopathic, and are related to underlying disease (**Box 1**), making

Table 1
The six determinants of gait

	First	Second	Third	Fourth and Fifth	Sixth
	Pelvic Rotation	Pelvic Tilt	Knee Flexion in Stance	Foot and Knee Mechanism	Lateral Displacement of the Pelvis
Activity	Rotation of 4° to each side	Tilt of 5° to each side	Knee flexes 15°	The ankle rotates at the heel in dorsiflexion while the knee is extended; then the ankle rotates at the forefoot in plantarflexion while the knee flexes	Tibiofemoral angle allows a relative adduction of the hip
Role	The combination of all determinants flattens the vertical and horizontal displacement of the COG				

Box 1
Medical conditions and risk factors associated with gait and balance disorders

Affective Disorders and Psychiatric Conditions

Depression

Fear of falling

Sleep disorders

Substance abuse

Infectious and Metabolic Diseases

Diabetes mellitus

Hepatic encephalopathy

Human immunodeficiency virus–associated neuropathy

Hyperthyroidism, hypothyroidism

Obesity

Tertiary syphilis

Uremia

Vitamin B_{12} deficiency

Neurologic Disorders

Cerebellar dysfunction or degeneration

Delirium

Dementia

Multiple sclerosis

Myelopathy

Normal-pressure hydrocephalus

Parkinson disease

Stroke

Vertebrobasilar insufficiency

Vestibular disorders

Cardiovascular Diseases

Arrhythmias

Congestive heart failure

Coronary artery disease

Orthostatic hypotension

Peripheral artery disease

Musculoskeletal Disorders

Cervical spondylosis

Gout

Lumbar spinal stenosis

Muscle weakness or atrophy

Osteoarthritis

Osteoporosis

Podiatric conditions

Sensory Abnormalities

Hearing impairment

Peripheral neuropathy

Visual impairment

Other

Acute medical illnesses

Recent hospitalizations

Recent surgery

Medications

the terms senile or normal inaccurate.[11,12] When declining gait patterns in aging are discussed, more attention should be given to making this distinction, considering establishing early identification of underlying disease, and taking prompt actions that could lead to preventive recommendations.

Reduced walking speed is the most consistent age-related change (**Box 2**). Gait speed of less than 1.0 m/s is considered abnormal, and spontaneous walking speed normally decreases by about 1% per year from age 60 years onward.[13,14] Gait speed less than 0.8 m/s is associated with limited capacity for community ambulation, whereas a gait speed equal to or slower than 0.4 m/s identifies people with an inability to meet basic ADLs.[15] Gait speed is considered a simple measure to screen for mobility changes, although some investigators do not consider it sensitive enough to detect early mobility decline. Speed of ambulation reflects efficiency, muscle strength, balance control, and endurance. To achieve this activity, several gait parameters play a key role: stride length, joint angular displacement, joint torque, and power. Ko and colleagues[16] described in a longitudinal study how older adults experienced a decline in speed and mediolateral hip control. Gait speed and stride

---

Box 2
Gait deviations associated with aging

Reduced walking speed

Decline in mediolateral hip control

Decreased stride length

Increased stride width

Increase in the stance phase

Reduced peak hip extension

Increased anterior pelvic tilt

Reduced-angle plantar flexion

Reduced hip motion

Decreased ambulation efficiency

Decreased muscle strength

Impaired balance control

length were significantly lower with increasing age.[16] This decline is more pronounced at fast walking speeds compared with usual speed. Stride width and the stance percentage of the gait cycle increased in the usually selected speed; patients spent more time of the cycle in hip flexion and ankle plantar flexion. Depending on the walking task (usual pace vs fast walking), elders may use different mechanical work expenditures (MWEs) in response or in compensation for limited joint rotation or weakness. Changes in MWE are not necessarily equivalent to metabolic energy consumption. In the case of the hip joint during usual speed walking, it seems to generate higher anteroposterior (AP) hip flexion MWE to compensate for speed when there is lower hip rotational motion. The opposite occurs in hip extension, in which the AP hip absorption MWE is reduced at the usual speed; this may imply a functional challenge during the critical weight-supporting phase. In the case of the ankle at fast speed walking, it manifests lower AP MWE during late-stance ankle plantar flexion moment, which may represent reduced ankle propulsion before swing, causing a shorter swing or problems with foot clearance. Ko and colleagues[16] described a lower range of hip and ankle rotation in the mediolateral plane in all walking tasks, as well as MWE. This finding can probably be attributed to lower angular speed and strength in the hip abductor group, and may be one of the core reasons for declining mobility performance in elders.

There are other alterations observed in the gait pattern, like reduced peak hip extension, increased anterior pelvic tilt, reduced ankle plantar flexion, and changed power generation. In the elderly, speed decline results from decrements in stride length and cadence, and loss of muscle strength. The muscle groups associated with this weakness are the same as are observed as protagonists in the gait cycle: ankle dorsiflexors, ankle plantarflexors, knee extensors, hip flexors, and hip extensors.[17]

Energy Cost

Routine physical activity accounts for 15% to 30% of adults' total daily energy expenditure, and walking is the most performed activity for most people. The walking energy cost in older adults is greater compared with younger adults, and this energetic cost has been related to self-reports of poor function in adults with mobility disability.[18] Theories explaining the energy cost are centered on biomechanical factors that impair the flow of ambulation. In a cross-sectional study performed by Wert and colleagues,[19] they were able to identify that lack of hip extension during walking explained a substantial proportion of the energy cost variance, followed by step width and cadence. Other investigators produced similar findings. Wert and colleagues[19] related energy cost to increased muscle demands associated with an increase cadence and work related to controlling the body's velocity and redirecting the limbs. Because the lack of hip extension produced higher energy cost, a comprehensive analysis was performed to understand the specifics of oxygen consumption (Vo_2) and energy reserves. This analysis showed that older adults with severe reduction of hip extension could walk with an energy cost close to the Vo_2 max (75%–87%), leaving only a minimal reserve of energy to perform other tasks. The authors invite readers to ponder the ability of elders to perform other functional activities with the remaining energy reserve.

Posture alterations also contribute to increased energy cost. Saha and colleagues[20] reported that there was increased O_2 consumption with increased trunk flexion. This finding was again attributed to work performed by muscles seeking to maintain an upright balance by supporting the head and trunk against gravity.[20]

Postural Changes

The posture of old adults is stereotyped as stooped. This positioning of the body includes forward head, kyphosis of the thoracic spine, and loss of the lumbar lordosis (**Fig. 4**). Other features that accompany this posturing are a wide base of support, slight knee flexion, and forward inclination of the trunk. To compensate for these changes, there is an increase in the hip flexion angle.[21]

Aging reduces postural stability, the efficiency of voluntary movement planning, in addition to negatively affecting the body's response planning.[22] Body postural changes are more commonly seen after the sixth decade, but symptoms and manifestations may begin as early as the fourth decade. Physical changes progress slowly and accelerate after the 60s, particularly in women. Contributing factors are known to be multifactorial, and among them are a decrement in the efficiency of central and peripheral neurons, a decrease in the skeletal mass and muscle tissue, weight loss, connective tissue fragility, reduction in muscle strength, and changes in ligaments and articular cartilage. Under this influence, passive and active stabilizers of the spine are vulnerable to the upright position and the weight load, which contribute to degenerative and deforming processes at the spine and the hip joints. Diminished muscle strength facilitates altered body biomechanics, which unknowingly leads

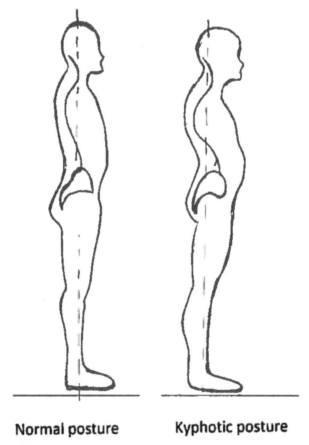

Normal posture   **Kyphotic posture**

Fig. 4. The kyphotic posture.

individuals into trying to balance in different postures, which keeps the cycle going, facilitating sustained structural changes. The outcome of these combined changes results in forward tilting of the trunk, which moves the COG forward. Functionally, this negatively influences the gait pattern, increases the risk for falls and disability, and diminishes the quality of life.[23]

MOBILITY PROBLEMS AND FUNCTIONAL INDEPENDENCE IN THE ELDERLY
Mobility and Activities of Daily Living

The most common risk factors for mobility impairment in patients are older age, low physical activity, obesity, strength or balance impairment, and chronic disease.[24] Mobility impairment leads to disability, which is known to have a higher prevalence among the older population compared with nonelderly groups. People move to perform ADLs, and when ADL measures deteriorate they can be significant predictors of admission to a nursing home, use of home care, use of hospital services, need for living arrangements, overall Medicare expenditures, insurance coverage, and mortality.[25]

Musculoskeletal pain is another reason for impaired balance and mobility problems, and it is considered to double the risk for mobility limitations.[26] The exact link between pain and mobility issues is not clearly described, but it is considered that pain limits physical activity, which consequently affects strength, which leads to the mobility limitation.

Gait speed by itself has been identified as an important predictor of onset of ADL disability.[2] Preferred or usual walking rates correlate with functional performance levels and activity. Patients who slow their walking speed are likely to decline in instrumental ADL (IADL) capacity. Studies suggest that the decline relates to body weakness, reduced capacity to execute controlled and coordinated body movements, or a lessened desire to engage in activities. Albert and colleagues[2] established that IADL disability threshold is between 0.8 and 0.6 m/s, which coincides with the findings of other investigators. Gait stability seems to be key for maintaining IADL abilities.[2] Cognitive function has been related to changes in gait speed, but has not been specifically studied in IADLs.

Muscle Strength

Muscle strength and balance are the impairments most commonly studied in mobility limitations. Weakness is described essentially in trunk and lower extremity muscles, specifically in trunk flexors and extensors, and in knee extensors[26] Rantanen and colleagues[27] associated lower extremity maximal isometric muscle strength with self-reported mobility difficulties, like walking outdoors and stair climbing. Other studies use hand grip strength thresholds to determine the likelihood of mobility limitation.[28]

Balance

Physical balance deteriorates with aging and leads to high risk for falls. The body uses control systems that collaborate to promote a stable gait and balance. These systems are the central nervous system (CNS), which allows delivery; the musculoskeletal system, for body maintenance and movement; the sensory system, for recurrent feedback of the movement; and vision, from which external information is acquired and used to manage uneven surfaces and promote dynamic stability. The most common gait strategy used to adapt to the external environment is slowing the gait speed, which increases the stance phase and, consequently, the physical stability. In the aging population, this environment adaptation is slow, and not necessarily achieved rapidly enough to attain body stability, which can lead to the risk for falls. Risk for falls can increase further because of environmental factors like low illumination. Compared with a younger population, the elderly do not seem to have the same ability to alter the gait pattern in response to dimly illuminated surfaces.[29]

Fear of Falling

Fear of falling is a well-studied factor that is related to mobility problems; it affects the mental and social life by influencing the self-confidence in the ability to walk safely. Tinetti and Powell[30] defined fear of falling as a lasting concern for falling, a perceived low self-confidence that leads individuals into avoiding activities that they remain capable of performing. This fear may affect the quality of life by limiting mobility, social interaction, sense of well-being, and quality of life. This sense of fear is not limited to the emotional and social component. Chamberlin and colleagues[31] described that the fear of falling influences spatial and temporal gait parameter changes in elderly persons. Specifically, they stated that, compared with fearless participants, fearful patients showed slower gait speed, shorter stride length, increased stride width, and prolonged double-limb support time.[31]

Other Independent Factors

Multiple coexisting impairments may have a greater impact on mobility decline because of the individual's inability to compensate for individual limitations.[32] Several investigators have addressed this question and have found that there is five times more risk for severe walking limitation if balance and strength are impaired compared with no impairment group, and three times more risk for severe walking limitation if balance was impaired even in the presence of good strength.[33]

CENTRAL NERVOUS SYSTEM, COGNITION, AND MOBILITY

Mahlknecht and colleagues[34] described in a population-based study that the prevalence of gait disorders is about 32%, and it increases with age. The CNS is a key contributor to mobility limitations, even in older adults who are free from neurologic disease. Studies can easily relate gait disorders when there is a CNS injury, but in cases in which there are subclinical CNS abnormalities, establishing this relationship has been more difficult. Most of the indirect evidence comes from older adults in whom gait is studied in relation to global cognitive abilities. The association becomes stronger when executive functions, including planning and coordination of a sequence of actions, are included in the equation. Changes in gait precede and predict cognitive decline, Alzheimer disease, vascular dementia, and stroke. In contrast, cognitive changes also negatively affect gait,[35] which may manifest as a difficulty in performing dual tasks, like walking and speaking at the same time. Structurally, these CNS abnormalities may be seen as generalized brain atrophy, small vessel disease, subclinical cerebral infarcts, Lewy bodies, neuritic plaques, neurofibrillary tangles, and white matter disease. These changes are not specific to mobility impairment, but are considered to adversely affect motor function and gait, and are common in older adults who do not have clinical neurologic disease.[36]

In addition to affecting gait markers, brain atrophy has been associated with decreased trunk stability during dual task performance, whereas the gray matter volume of the primary sensorimotor and medial temporal areas has been associated with bradykinesia and gait disturbance.

There are studies that suggest that exercise and environmental stimulation may activate brain plasticity that leads to neuronal remodeling. Similarly, it has been observed that physical activity can improve cognitive function and enhance brain structures, as well as that cognitive training can improve gait speed.[10]

Even when many gaps in knowledge have been identified, precise estimates of CNS contribution to gait impairment is therefore lacking, brain neuropathology and the underlying mechanism that leads to gait impairment are not clearly understood, and not all CNS disorders can be used to explain gait impairments. To close some of these gaps, researchers are challenged to study gait and mobility at an earlier stage in life, and longitudinally. Neuroimaging will play a key role in the future of understanding the structural changes in mechanism associated with gait.

GAPS IN EVIDENCE

Gait and mobility seem to be of interest to the research community. However, there are knowledge gaps with potential for future investigations. Some of these are longitudinal studies on the impact of metabolic energy consumption on gait in the elderly, functional MRI while performing ambulation, more neuroimaging studies of the structural brain changes and how they related to gait, gait changes in the aging under muscle fatigue conditions, and the effect that pain has on gait parameters in older adults.

SUMMARY

There are normal physiologic changes that occur as people age. Gait and mobility are altered with aging, and these changes are a combination of alterations in the gait pattern and in the function of organs. Changes in gait are associated with functional decline, less independence, and impaired quality of life. Reduced walking speed is the most consistent age-related change, but there are other contributors to an altered gait: impaired balance and stability, lower extremity strength, and fear of falling.

REFERENCES

1. Rughwani N. Normal anatomic and physiologic changes with aging and related disease outcomes: a refresher. Mt Sinai J Med 2011;78:509–14.
2. Albert SM, Bear-Lehman J, Anderson SJ. Declines in mobility and changes in performance in the instrumental activities of daily living among mildly disabled community-dwelling older adults. J Gerontol A Biol Sci Med Sci 2015;70(1):71–7.
3. Nutt JG, Marsden CD, Thompson PD. Human walking and higher level gait disorders, particularly in the elderly. Neurology 1993;43:268–79.
4. Cailliet R. The illustrated guide to functional anatomy of the musculoskeletal system. 2004.
5. Patla AE, Ishac MG, Winter DA. Anticipatory control of center of mass and joint stability during voluntary arm movement from a standing posture: interplay between active and passive control. Exp Brain Res 2002;143(3):318–27.
6. Berger N, Fishman S, editors. Normal gait. Lower limb prosthetics. New York: Prosthetic-Orthotic Publications; 1997. p. 15–32.
7. Saunders JB, Inman VT, Eberhart HD. The major determinants in normal and pathological gait. J Bone Joint Surg 1953;35A(3):543–58.
8. Sutherland DH, Olshen R, Copper L, et al. The development of mature gait. J Bone Joint Surg Am. 1980;62:336–53.

9. Verghese J, Levalley A, Hall CB, et al. Epidemiology of gait disorders in community-residing older adults. J Am Geriatr Soc 2006;54:255–61.

10. Sudarsky L. Gait disorders: prevalence, morbidity and etiology. Adv Neurol 2001; 87:111–7.

11. Salzman B. Gait and balance disorders in older adults. Am Fam Physician 2010; 82(1):61–8.

12. Jahn K, Zwergal A, Schniepp R. Gait disturbance in old age. Dtsch Arztebl Int 2010;107(17):306–16.

13. Ashton-Miller JA. Age-associated changes in the biomechanics of gait and gait-related falls in older adults. In: Hausdorff JM, Alexander NB, editors. Gait disorders: evaluation and management. Boca Raton (FL): Taylor & Francis; 2005. p. 63–100.

14. Brach JS, Perera S, VanSwearingen JM, et al. Challenging gait conditions predict 1-year decline in gait speed in older adults with apparently normal gait. Phys Ther 2011;91(12):1857–64.

15. Fritz S, Lusardi M. White paper: "Walking speed: the sixth vital sign". J Geriatr Phys Ther 2009;32(2):46–9.

16. Ko SU, Hausdorff JM, Ferrucci L. Age-associated differences in the gait. Age Ageing 2010;39(6):688–94.

17. Pease WS, Bowyer BL, Kadyan V. Human walking. In: Delisa JA, Their SO, editors. Physical medicine & rehabilitation: principles & practice. 4th edition. Lippincott Williams & Wilkins; 2005. p. 155–68.

18. Wert DM, BJ, VanSwearingen J. Energy cost of walking contributes to physical function in older adults. In: American Geriatrics Society Annual Conference. 2009 Annual Scientific Meeting Abstract Book. Vol. 57(4). Chicago: Wiley-Blackwell; 2009.

19. Wert DM, Brach J, Perera S, et al. Gait biomechanics, spatial and temporal characteristics, and the energy cost of walking in older adults with impaired mobility. Phys Ther 2010;90(7):977–85.

20. Saha D, Gard S, Fatone S, et al. The effect of trunk-flexed postures on balance and metabolic energy expenditure during standing. Spine 2007;32:1605–11.

21. Hayes C. Ambulation in older people – mobility explained. Br J Healthc Assistants 2014;08(3):124–9.

22. Rubenstein LZ. Falls in older people: epidemiology, risk factors and strategies for prevention. Age an Ageing 2006;35(Suppl 2):ii37–41.

23. Drzał-Grabiec J, Snela S, Rykała J, et al. Changes in the body posture of women occurring with age. BMC Geriatr 2013;13:108.

24. Brown CJ, Flood KL. Mobility limitation in the older patient: a clinical review. JAMA 2013;310(11):1168–77.

25. Wiener JM, Hanley RJ. Measuring the activities of daily living among the elderly: a guide to national surveys. US Department of Health and Human Services; 1989.

26. Rantakokko M, Mänty M, Rantanen T. Mobility decline in old age. Exerc Sport Sci Rev 2013;41(1):19–25.

27. Rantanen T, Era P, Heikkinen E. Maximal isometric strength and mobility among 75-year-old men and women. Age Ageing 1994;23(2):132–7.

28. Sallinen J, Stenholm S, Rantanen T, et al. Hand-grip strength cut points to screen older persons at risk for mobility limitation. J Am Geriatr Soc 2010;58(9):1721–6.

29. Choi JS, Kang DW, Shin YH, et al. Differences in gait pattern between the elderly and the young during level walking under low illumination. Acta Bioeng Biomech 2014;16(1):3–9.

30. Tinetti M, Powell L. Fear of falling and low self-efficacy: a cause of dependence in elderly persons. J Gerontol 1993;48:35–8.

31. Chamberlin ME, Fulwider BD, Sanders SL, et al. Does fear of falling influence spatial and temporal gait parameters in elderly persons beyond changes associated with normal aging? J Gerontol A Biol Sci Med Sci 2005;60A(9):1163–7.

32. Rantanen T, Guralnik JM, Ferrucci L, et al. Coimpairments: strength and balance as predictors of severe walking disability. J Gerontol A Biol Sci Med Sci 1999; 54(4):M172–6.

33. Rantanen T, Guralnik JM, Ferrucci L, et al. Coimpairments as predictors of severe walking disability in older women. J Am Geriatr Soc 2001;49(1):21–7.

34. Mahlknecht P, Kiechl S, Bloem BR, et al. Prevalence and burden of gait disorders in elderly men and women aged 60–97 years: a population-based study. PLoS One 2013;8(7):e69627.

35. Rosso AL, Studenski SA, Chen WG, et al. Aging, the central nervous system, and mobility. J Gerontol A Biol Sci Med Sci 2013;68(11):1379–86.

36. Holtzer R, Epstein N, Mahoney JR, et al. Neuroimaging of mobility in aging: a targeted review. J Gerontol A Biol Sci Med Sci 2014;69(11):1375–88.

Balance Problems and Fall Risks in the Elderly

Ramon Cuevas-Trisan, MD

KEYWORDS

- Balance • Falls • Older adults • Risk factors

KEY POINTS

- Fall prevention strategies are important interventions in all elderly individuals.
- Prevention of falls can decrease morbidity and mortality in the elderly.
- Evaluation and effective intervention strategies are generally multifactorial.

INTRODUCTION
Demographics and Scope of the Problem

Falls are an important cause of morbidity and mortality and the leading cause of fatal and nonfatal injuries among older adults. According to data obtained from the Behavioral Risk Factor Surveillance System survey and analyzed by the Centers for Disease Control and Prevention, in 2014, approximately 28.7% of older adults reported falling at least once in the preceding 12 months, resulting in an estimated 29.0 million falls and 7.0 million fall injuries in the United States.[1] Injury severity varies but 2.8 million were treated in emergency departments for fall-related injuries and approximately 800,000 of these individuals were subsequently hospitalized. Of those who fell, 37.5% reported at least one fall that required medical treatment or restricted activity for at least 1 day.[1] Approximately 27,000 older adults died because of falls during that same period.

Women are more likely to report falling and to report a fall injury than men. The percentage of older adults who fall increases with age, from 26.7% among persons aged 65 to 74 years, to 29.8% among persons aged 75 to 84 years, to 36.5% among persons aged greater than or equal to 85 years.[2] It is generally known that falling in the elderly is usually caused by various factors. Therefore, multifactorial interventions may be more effective than any one single intervention.

Disclosures: The author has nothing to disclose.
Physical Medicine and Rehabilitation Service, West Palm Beach VA Medical Center, University of Miami Miller School of Medicine, Nova Southeastern University College of Osteopathic Medicine, 7305 North Military Trail, PM&RS (117), West Palm Beach, FL 33410-6400, USA
E-mail address: ramon.cuevas-trisan@va.gov

Phys Med Rehabil Clin N Am 28 (2017) 727–737
http://dx.doi.org/10.1016/j.pmr.2017.06.006
1047-9651/17/Published by Elsevier Inc.
pmr.theclinics.com

PATIENT ASSESSMENT
Conditions

***
Gait and balance disorders
Gait and balance disorders are among the most common causes of falls in older adults and often lead to injury, disability, loss of independence, and limitations in quality of life. Good balance is likely a rapid synergistic interaction between various physiologic and cognitive elements that allow rapid and precise response to a perturbation.[3] It is a remarkable complex relationship between systems that allow for rapid and precise changes to prevent a fall (concept of reaction time). Gait and balance disorders are usually multifactorial in origin and require a comprehensive assessment to determine contributing factors and targeted interventions. Most changes in gait occurring in older adults are related to underlying medical conditions, particularly as conditions increase in severity, and should not be viewed as merely an inevitable consequence of aging. Early identification of gait and balance disorders and appropriate intervention may prevent dysfunction and loss of independence.[4] The prevalence of abnormal gait increases with age and is higher in persons in the acute hospital setting and in those living in long-term care facilities.

Cognitive impairment
Neurocognitive functions powerfully influence fall risk.[5] Cognitive impairment, regardless of the diagnosis, is a risk factor for falls.[6] Cognitively impaired adults show an increased risk of falls compared with their age-matched cognitively intact peers.[7] The increasing incidence of various forms of dementia and degrees of cognitive impairment in older adults has increased the prevalence of falls in this population.[8]

Early fall prevention in adults with mild cognitive problems follows a strong rationale. This population is at high risk of functional decline and generally has significant comorbidities. Falls can contribute to this decline through injury, hospital admission, loss of confidence, and deconditioning from reduced activity. Any intervention that can reduce the risk of future falls at an early stage has the potential to maintain function and activity level, thus reducing the progression into disability and dependency. By helping people to adopt techniques to stay healthy (ie, strength and balance exercises) and adaptations that reduce risk (ie, appropriate mobility aids, home hazard reduction) at an early stage of cognitive impairment, these practices could theoretically help as cognitive decline progresses.[8] Cognitive assessment is strongly advised but there is no clear guidance on how to respond to individuals with cognitive impairment because recommendations and evidence for effective fall prevention interventions for older adults with cognitive impairment are not well documented.[9]

Musculoskeletal conditions and pain
Persistent pain, impaired mobility and function, and reduced quality of life are the most common experiences associated with musculoskeletal conditions. The prevalence and impact of musculoskeletal conditions increase with aging. Population growth, aging, and sedentary lifestyles, particularly in developing countries, have created a crisis for population health that requires a multisystem response with musculoskeletal health services as a critical component. Globally, there is an emphasis on maintaining an active lifestyle to fight numerous ailments associated with sedentary habits. However, painful musculoskeletal conditions profoundly limit the ability of people to make these lifestyle changes. A strong relationship exists between painful musculoskeletal conditions and a reduced capacity to engage in physical activity resulting in functional decline, frailty, reduced well-being, and loss of independence. In a group of community-dwelling adults older than 88 years in the Netherlands, joint pain was

reported as the most common contributor to gait problems, followed by several other causes.[10] The use of mobility aids (eg, various types of canes and walkers) can help with stability and help reduce the contribution of musculoskeletal problems to falls. These, however, must be properly adjusted or fitted for the individual to effectively help unload painful joints. Additionally, when improperly prescribed, these could result in the patients not using them or worse yet, contribute to increase the incidence of falls.[11] Many physiatric therapies and interventions are available to address the negative impact of musculoskeletal conditions.

Vision

Visual impairment is an underrepresented area of research for falls among older adults but is generally recognized to be an important risk factor. The prevalence of vision impairment and blindness increases with age and poor vision as a risk factor for falls is sometimes overlooked because the process of decreasing vision is often slow and may even be unnoticeable for some older individuals. Impaired visual acuity increases the risk of falls and injuries, and bilateral visual field loss caused by glaucoma is associated with greater fear of falling with an impact that exceeds numerous other risk factors.[12]

Improving visual function may have benefits, such as decreased traumatic events and improved mobility. However, changes should be made with caution because well-meaning and rational interventions can increase the risk of falls (a study found that the falling rate of the visually intervened was higher than in the control group).[13] One possible explanation is that improved vision may lead to changes in behavior that increase exposure to fall-pone situations. Additionally, vision-related interventions tend to focus on correcting central vision when both central and peripheral vision components may be necessary to effectively reduce rates of falls.[12] Investigators analyzed data from seven high-quality studies evaluating visual problems as risk factors targeting interventions for visual loss. They identified various combinations of targeted interventions in the setting of visual impairment and concluded that visual intervention plus various risk factor assessments and interventions were more effective than visual intervention alone or other combined interventions (eg, exercise and vision) in preventing falls in older people.[12] A Cochrane review on the subject also revealed that first eye cataract surgery reduces the rate of falls.[11]

Medications

The use of multiple medications (four or more), and specific classes of medications, can lead to gait and balance disorders and increased rate of falls.[14,15] The concept of medication reconciliation (the process of reviewing all the medications that a patient is taking prescribed by any and all providers) has gained importance and is increasingly being used in all clinical settings. It has long been recognized that polypharmacy is a source of many iatrogenic problems, from side effects caused by drug-drug interactions to continuation of unnecessary medications. Providers need to recognize that many medications, especially those with central nervous system effects, need to be used with caution in elderly individuals because of the effects that these could have altering their reaction time, memory, balance, and brain perfusion. Notable offenders include opioids, benzodiazepines, diuretics, vasodilators, tricyclic antidepressants, skeletal muscle relaxants, β-blockers, antihistamine medications, and sleep aids. Antiplatelet agents and anticoagulants, common in the elderly because of associated cardiovascular ailments, add another layer of complexity, potentially making falls catastrophic.

The practice of managing medication side effects with other medications, although common in the clinical setting, is rarely justified and physicians should always consider discontinuing and replacing the original medication before adding another to treat undesirable side effects.

Sarcopenia

Sarcopenia is a syndrome characterized by progressive and generalized loss of skeletal muscle mass and strength with a risk of adverse outcomes, such as physical disability, poor quality of life, and death.[16] Its precise diagnostic criteria and pathophysiology are beyond the scope of this article but its prevalence, which may be 30% for those older than 60 years of age, will increase as the percentage of the very old continues to grow.[17] Sarcopenia and physical frailty run along the same continuum. Physical frailty in its initial phase can still be reversed and fighting sarcopenia in elderly persons has the potential to slow or halt the progressive decline toward disability and dependency.

Box 1 provides an overview of potential causes for falls in older adults. The clinician should consider assessing for fall risk when any of these conditions are present.

Patient Evaluation

History

The patient's history should include specific questions about known risk factors for falls. It is imperative to ask about prior falls and the circumstances surrounding these, because patients who have fallen in the last year are significantly more likely to fall again (likelihood ratio, 2.3–2.8).[18]

The clinician should always inquire about environmental hazards. Some common hazards include poor lighting, rugs, areas of high clutter, electrical cords, slippery surfaces, steps, and stairways. Whenever possible, the clinician should include other family members in this conversation because patients tend to downplay the importance of some of these hazards. A functional history should always be obtained including ability to perform basic and instrumental activities of daily living.[4]

Physical examination

Inspection for joint deformities, swelling, and bruises is an important component of the examination. Joint instability and passive and active range of motion limitations in the major joints of the lower limb joints and spine should be evaluated, including assessing for soft tissue tightness that may produce limitations. Commonly encountered problems include tight hamstrings and tight iliopsoas, limiting knee and hip extension, respectively. These limitations alter the normal gait pattern and in turn the body's center of gravity, contributing to greater energy consumption during the gait cycle and balance challenges.

Posture, particularly excess kyphosis commonly seen in older persons, can significantly shift the body's center of gravity. Forward shift of the head with limited neck extension also alters the center of gravity and contributes to postural imbalance and limits the functional peripheral visual field.

Ideal footwear should fit properly, be comfortable (taking into account common foot deformities, such as hallux valgus and per cavus), provide wide support and stability, and be lightweight for ease during foot advancement.

A focused neurologic examination to detect deficits, such as sensory impairments (particularly proprioception), and weakness should always be performed because it may reveal potentially treatable problems. Proprioceptive impairment caused by a neuropathy, for example, is a common cause of balance impairment in older adults. Decreased vibration sense, a frequent but abnormal finding in this population, is a more sensitive marker of neuropathy than a decrease in position sense. Balance

Box 1
Risk factors associated with gait and balance disorders in the older adult

Neurologic disorders

Delirium/dementia

Cerebellar dysfunction

Myelopathy

Normal pressure hydrocephalus

Stroke

Parkinson's disease and related disorders

Peripheral neuropathies

Visual impairment

Myopathies

Cardiovascular disorders

Congestive heart failure

Arrhythmias

Peripheral arterial disease

Orthostatic hypotension

Musculoskeletal disorders

Spinal stenosis

Painful arthritides/spondylosis

Lower limb deformities

Muscle weakness and atrophy (sarcopenia)

Other medical disorders

Most acute medical illnesses

Medications: diuretics, opioids, benzodiazepines, anticonvulsants, antidepressants, psychotropics, anticholinergics, sleep aids

Obesity

Vitamin B_{12} deficiency

Diabetes

Uremia

Hepatic encephalopathy

Substance use disorders

This list is not comprehensive, but provides an overview of potential causes. The clinician should consider assessing for fall risk when any of these conditions are present.

that worsens with the eyes closed and improves when minor support is given by the examiner is another clue for proprioceptive problems.[19] Additionally, the clinician should assess for coordination, tone, tremors, cognition, and depression (usually with a validated questionnaire).

Evaluation of gait is an essential step to identify persons at fall risk. Observational gait assessment should assess velocity, stride length, antalgic movements, balance, stance, and symmetry. If it seems normal and functional, challenges should be introduced by asking the individual to walk on toes and heels. Tandem and backward walking, and unipedal stance, are particularly useful tests for detection of more subtle balance problems. These should be performed carefully and the clinician should be prepared to provide physical assistance if needed during testing to prevent a fall.

Observational ability to get up from a chair is also an excellent screening for function, testing proximal strength, balance, and coordination simultaneously. Other formal functional tests, such as the Timed Up and Go Test, are reliable and easy to administer. Such tests as the Berg Balance Scale and the Performance-Oriented Mobility Assessment are excellent but more time consuming. The Functional Reach Test is another reliable, valid, and quick diagnostic test for postural stability.[4] The general evaluation is not complete without obtaining the vital signs with particular attention to possible orthostatic hypotension, along with screenings for hearing and visual problems. Cardiovascular conditions are highly prevalent in older adults. Certain arrhythmias can lead to syncope and falls. A Cochrane database review concluded that pacemakers reduced the rate of falls in people with carotid sinus hypersensitivity.[11] When assessed appropriately, clinically significant postural hypotension is detected in up to 30% of elderly persons but unfortunately, some elderly persons with postural hypotension do not report symptoms, such as dizziness or lightheadedness.[19] **Fig. 1** provides an outline of the key components of the physical examination for an older adult at risk for falls. **Table 1** provides symptoms and signs and associated selected disorders causing decreased balance and falls in the older adult.

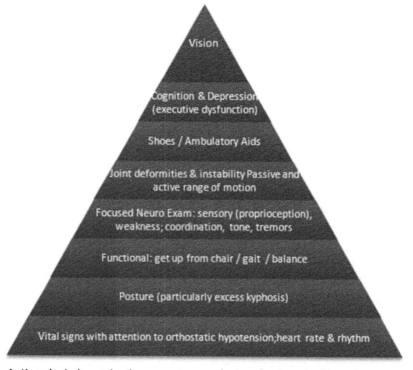

Fig. 1. Key physical examination components when evaluating an older adult for risk of falling.

Table 1
Symptoms and signs and associated disorders affecting gait/balance

Signs/Symptoms	Associated Disorders
Back pain, claudication (worsens with extension improved with flexion)	Spinal stenosis
Hyperreflexia, imbalance, spasticity	Myelopathy, stroke
Mixed upper/lower motor neuron findings	Vitamin B_{12} deficiency
Trunk instability, wide base gait, ataxia	Cerebellar disease
Tremor, rigidity, bradykinesia	Parkinson's disease
Proximal weakness	Myopathies, PMR
Sensory deficits, acroparesthesias	Peripheral neuropathies
Cognitive impairment, poor judgment	Dementia (AD, others)
Focal motor/sensory deficits, cognitive decline	Vascular dementia, stroke
Memory loss, ataxia, urinary incontinence	Normal pressure hydrocephalus
History of falls with head trauma	SDH
Kyphosis	VCFs, camptocormia
Decreased ROM, joint deformities	Degenerative joint disease
Visual impairment	Glaucoma (peripheral), cataracts (blurred), macular degeneration (central)
Palpitations, chest pain, DOE	CHF, CAD, arrhythmias
Dizziness, vertigo	Vestibular problems, medication S/E
Drop attacks (sudden falls without dizziness/vertigo)	Vertebrobasilar insufficiency, seizures
Lightheadedness with sudden head turning	Carotid sinus hypersensitivity
Lightheadedness with sudden rise	Orthostatic hypotension (medication S/E)

Abbreviations: AD, Alzheimer disease; CAD, coronary artery disease; CHF, congestive heart failure; DOE, dyspnea on exertion; PMR, polymyalgia rheumatica; ROM, range of motion; S/E, side effects; SDH, subdural hematoma; VCF, vertebral compression fractures.

PREVENTION AND MANAGEMENT STRATEGIES
Nonpharmacologic

Exercise
The recommendations and general benefits of exercise in the older adult would generally include the incorporation of activities that maintain or increase flexibility, endurance, strength, and balance. In addition, an older adult with a medical condition for which exercise is therapeutic should perform exercises in a manner that treats the condition and should engage in physical activity in a manner that reduces the risk of developing other chronic diseases. Exercise plans should include a gradual (stepwise) approach to increase physical activity over time.[20] Muscle strengthening and weight-bearing activities are particularly important in the older adult given their role in preventing age-related loss of muscle mass, bone, and functional abilities.[20]

Meta-analyses have shown that exercising has consistent effects reducing falls in healthy older adult populations when prescribed and completed at the correct progression and intensity.[21,22] A 2009 Cochrane database review concluded that multiple-component group exercise programs reduced the rate of falls and risk of falling, as did Tai Chi and individually prescribed multiple-component home-based exercise programs.[11] A more recent meta-analysis concluded that exercise reduced the rate of falls in community-dwelling older people by 21%, with greater effects seen from exercise programs that challenged balance and involved more than 3 h/wk of duration. The investigators also found that exercise had a fall prevention effect in community-dwelling people with Parkinson's disease or cognitive impairment but no evidence of a fall prevention effect of exercise in residential care settings, among stroke survivors, or people recently discharged from the hospital.[21–23]

Masakazu and colleagues[24] compared the frequency of falls among 91 institutionalized frail elderly residents following three different interventions: (1) low-frequency exercise, (2) vitamin D supplementation, and (3) a combination of both. The intervention combining low-frequency exercise and vitamin D supplementation was the most effective for the reduction of falls among institutionalized frail elderly individuals.

From the public health and population management perspective, experts from Korea, Hong Kong, Taiwan, and Australia presented their research during the International Association of Gerontology and Geriatrics World Congress in Seoul (June 2013).[25] Meta-analyses presented revealed that in the elderly, Tai Chi is beneficial for balance improvement, and can lead to fall reductions (based on 13 randomized controlled trials). They recommended that communities should establish effective fall prevention programs; that exercise programs are an effective single prevention strategy; that environmental modifications are effective; and that multifactorial interventions, including exercise programs, can be recommended despite the need for more research.[25]

Specific exercise targets include strength, endurance, flexibility, and balance. A Cochrane review evaluating outcomes of these interventions revealed that programs targeting at least two of these components reduce the rate of falls. Furthermore, group exercises, such as Tai Chi and individually prescribed home exercise programs, are also effective. The role of physical therapy in targeting these strategies cannot be overstated.[11]

Environmental assessments and modifications

Environmental assessment and modification has proven to be effective preventing falls in community-dwelling older people. The training, experience, and approach of the individual performing the assessment and providing the recommendations are important factors in their effectiveness.[26]

Although nonspecific advice about modification of home hazards directed at untargeted groups of elderly persons has not been proven effective, standardized assessment of home hazards by an occupational therapist, along with specific recommendations and follow-up after hospital discharge, was associated with a 20% reduction in the risk of falling.[11,27] The most commonly recommended modifications in that study were the removal of rugs, a change to safer footwear, the use of nonslip bathmats, the use of lighting at night, and the addition of stair rails.[19] Evidence strongly supports the assessment and modification of the patient's home environment as part of a multifactorial fall prevention program, being particularly beneficial in high-risk individuals, such as those with prior history of falls.[11]

Pharmacologic

The concept of medication reconciliation and medication burden reduction has finally become standard of practice. Polypharmacy is commonplace in the elderly and it is not uncommon for patients to be treated by multiple medical providers with little to no coordination of care. Therefore, it is common to see medications prescribed to address side effects from other medications, resulting in a wide variety of problematic side effects and a large number of clinically important drug-drug interactions. Some common side effects include orthostatic hypotension, dizziness, and somnolence, all of which have been associated with falls. In one study, tapering and discontinuation of psychotropic medications, including benzodiazepines, other sleep medications, neuroleptic agents, and antidepressants, over a 14-week period was associated with a 39% reduction in the rate of falling.[28] Successful components of these interventions include review and possible reduction of medications.

SUMMARY

The clinical relevance of the multifactorial relationships of the deficits that lead to falls in older adults is that improvement in modifiable factors may help compensate for those functions or factors that are irreversibly affected.[3] Known effective strategies for reducing the number of older adult falls call for a multifactorial clinical approach, including gait and balance assessment, strength and balance exercises, environmental modifications, and medication review.[1] Implementing these on a large scale can prove to be challenging, as documented by investigators from the State Falls Prevention Project, a project funded by the Centers for Disease Control and Prevention, in which several state Departments of Health were charged with implementing clinical and community fall-prevention programs in specific geographic areas. Some of the challenges that they identified include difficulties and resistance to change physician practice, lack of program availability in many communities coupled with limited knowledge about their availability and value (when available), and long-term sustainability of these programs.[29]

Although there is no consensus about the optimal time to initiate screening, the rate of falling and the prevalence of risk factors for falling increase steeply after the age of 70 years.[2,30,31] Guidelines from several professional societies recommend that all elderly patients should be asked about any falls that have occurred during the previous year and should undergo clinical screenings of their gait and balance.[32] Health care providers play a crucial role in fall prevention by screening older adults for fall risk, reviewing and managing medications linked to falls, and recommending preventive strategies.

REFERENCES

1. Bergen G, Stevens MR, Burns ER. Falls and fall injuries among adults aged $\geq$ 65 years—United States, 2014. MMWR Morb Mortal Wkly Rep 2016;65(37):993–8.
2. Nevitt MC, Cummings SR, Hudes ES. Risk factors for injurious falls: a prospective study. J Gerontol 1991;46:M164–70.
3. Richardson JK. The confusing circular nature of falls research… and a possible antidote. Am J Phys Med Rehabil 2017;96:55–9.
4. Salzman B. Gait and balance disorders in older adults. Am Fam Physician 2010; 82(1):61–8.
5. Kearney FC, Harwood RH, Gladman JR, et al. The relationship between executive function and falls and gait abnormalities in older adults: a systematic review. Dement Geriatr Cogn Disord 2013;36:20–35.
6. Lord SR, Sherrington C, Menz HB, et al. Falls in older people: risk factors and strategies for prevention. Cambridge (United Kingdom): Cambridge University Press; 2007.
7. Shaw FE, Bond J, Richardson DA, et al. Multifactorial intervention after a fall in older people with cognitive impairment and dementia presenting to the accident and emergency department: randomised controlled trial. BMJ 2003; 326:73.

8. Booth V, Harwood R, Hood V, et al. Understanding the theoretical underpinning of the exercise component in a fall prevention programme for older adults with mild dementia: a realist review protocol. Syst Rev 2016;5:119.

9. NICE. Clinical Guideline 161. Falls: assessment and prevention of falls in older people. Available at: https://www.nice.org.uk/guidance/cg161. Accessed December 19, 2014.

10. Bloem BR, Haan J, Lagaay AM, et al. Investigation of gait in elderly subjects over 88 years of age. J Geriatr Psychiatry Neurol 1992;5(2):78–84.

11. Gillespie LD, Gillespie WJ, Robertson MC, et al. Interventions for preventing falls in elderly people. Cochrane Database Syst Rev 2009;(2):CD000340.

12. Zhang X-Y, Shuai J, Li L-P. Vision and relevant risk factor interventions for preventing falls among older people: a network meta-analysis. Sci Rep 2015;5:10559.

13. Grue EV, Kirkevold M, Mowinchel P, et al. Sensory impairment in hip fracture patients 65 years or older and effects of hearing/vision interventions on fall frequency. J Multidisc Healthcare 2008;2:1–11.

14. Leipzig RM, Cummin RG, Tineti ME. Drugs and falls in older people: a systematic review and meta-analysis: I. Psychotropic drugs. J Am Geriatr Soc 1999;47(1):30–9.

15. Leipzig RM, Cummin RG, Tineti ME. Drugs and falls in older people: a systematic review and meta-analysis: II. Cardiac and analgesic drugs. J Am Geriatr Soc 1999;47(1):40–50.

16. Delmonico MJ, Harris TB, Lee JS, et al. Alternative definitions of sarcopenia, lower extremity performance, and functional impairment with aging in older men and women. J Am Geriatr Soc 2007;55:769–74.

17. Doherty TJ. Aging and sarcopenia (invited review). J Appl Physiol 2003;95(4):1717–27.

18. Ganz DA, Bao Y, Shekelle PG, et al. Will my patient fall? JAMA 2007;297(1):77–86.

19. Tinetti ME. Preventing falls in elderly persons. N Engl J Med 2003;348:42–9.

20. Nelson ME, Rejeski WJ, Blair SN, et al. Physical activity and public health in older adults. recommendation from the American College of Sports Medicine and the American Heart Association. Circulation 2007;116:1094–105.

21. Sherrington C, Michaleff ZA, Fairhall N, et al. Exercise to prevent falls in older adults: an updated systematic review and meta-analysis. Br J Sports Med 2016. http://dx.doi.org/10.1136/bjsports-2016-096547.

22. Sherrington C, Tiedemann A, Fairhall N, et al. Exercise to prevent falls in older adults: an updated meta-analysis and best practice recommendations. N S W Public Health Bull 2011;22(4):78–83.

23. Sherrington C, Tiedemann A, Fairhall NJ, et al. Exercise for preventing falls in older people living in the community. Cochrane Database Syst Rev 2016;(11):CD012424.

24. Masakazu I, Higuchi Y, Todo E, et al. Low-frequency exercise and Vitamin D supplementation reduce falls among institutionalized frail elderly. Intl J Geront 2016;1–5.

25. Kim EJ, Arai H, Chan P, et al. Strategies on fall prevention for older people living in the community: a report from a round-table meeting in IAGG 2013. J Clin Geront Geriatr 2015;6:39–44.

26. Pighills A, Ballinger A, Pickering R, et al. A critical review of the effectiveness of environmental assessment and modification in the prevention of falls amongst community dwelling older people. Br J Occup Ther 2015;79(3):133–43.

27. Cummings RG, Thomas M, Szonyi G, et al. Home visits by an occupational therapist for assessment and modification of environmental hazards: a randomized trial of falls prevention. J Am Geriatr Soc 1999;47:1397–402.

28. Campbell AJ, Robertson MC, Gardner MM, et al. Psychotropic medication withdrawal and a homebased exercise program to prevent falls: a randomized, controlled trial. J Am Geriatr Soc 1999;47:850–3.

29. Shubert TE, Smith ML, Schneider EC, et al. Commentary: public health system perspective on implementation of evidence-based fall-prevention strategies for older adults. Front Public Health 2016;4:252.

30. Nevitt MC, Cummings SR, Kidd S, et al. Risk factors for recurrent non-syncopal falls: a prospective study. JAMA 1989;261:2663–8.

31. Sattin RW. Falls among older persons: a public health perspective. Annu Rev Public Health 1992;13:489–508.

32. American Geriatrics Society, British Geriatric Society, American Academy of Orthopaedic Surgeons Panel on Falls Prevention. Guideline for the prevention of falls in older persons. J Am Geriatr Soc 2001;49:664–72.

Clinical Pharmacology and the Risks of Polypharmacy in the Geriatric Patient

Jose Luis Pesante-Pinto, MD

KEYWORDS

- Clinical pharmacology • Polypharmacy risk • Geriatric patient

KEY POINTS

- The elderly population is increasing globally in proportion as well as lifespan.
- Despite the fact that normal aging leads to physiologic changes, these patients encounter different threats, most of which are susceptible to medical interventions.
- Widespread use of prescription drugs in this frail group of patients is a hazard for the individual and collective life.
- Many of these threats are preventable.
- The judicious use of early management strategies and interventions is recommended.

INTRODUCTION
Impact of Aging Population

The World Health Organization estimates that worldwide, the proportion of older people in the total population is increasing at more than 3 times the overall population growth rate, and before 2020, the population of people age 65 and older will outnumber children under age 5. Americans are living longer and healthier lives. According to the Centers for Disease Control and Prevention (CDC) for the United States the Healthy Life Expectancy (HALE) at birth on 2015 was 69.1 years for both sexes, with an increase of about 2 years since 2000 (67.2 years). Using maximum-reported age-at-death data, the Albert Einstein School of Medicine researchers put the average maximum human life span at 115 years.[1]

The normal aging process

The normal aging process is characterized by a progression of physiologic changes affecting the body throughout the life cycle, and is more evident in the later years.

Disclosure Statement: The author has nothing to disclose.
Family Medicine Department, Universidad Central del Caribe School of Medicine, PO Box 60327, Bayamón, PR 00960-6032, USA
E-mail address: jose.pesante@uccaribe.edu

Phys Med Rehabil Clin N Am 28 (2017) 739–746
http://dx.doi.org/10.1016/j.pmr.2017.06.007

Every older person ages at his or her own physiologic or organic pace, in his or her unique circumstance based on his or her changing history.

During this period throughout the life cycle, the older adult encounters different threats, most of them susceptible to medical interventions, either prevention or management. One example of this is related with smoking. A study published in 2012 by the CDC about mortality drivers of trends in the older population found that the reduction of smoking at a younger age is expected to improve survivorship for these cohorts when they reach the older ages (population aged 64–83 years in 2050).[2]

Geriatric Syndromes

Despite those projections and preventive interventions, many older adults develop what is known as geriatric syndromes, which are problems that usually have more than 1 cause and involve many parts of the body, resulting in reduced quality of life and quantitative reduction in age.

In the older adult, geriatrics syndrome is a poorly defined concept that comprises clinical conditions and problems in different organs and parts of the body that cannot be classified as specific diseases. Many of these problems include elder frailty, falls, urinary incontinence, dizziness, syncope, and cognitive impairment.

Frailty syndrome

Frailty syndrome require as least 3 of the following 5 characteristics:

- Unintentional weight loss, as evidenced by a loss of at least 10 pounds or greater than 5% of body weight in the prior year; this occurs in 15% to 20% of older adults and is associated with increased morbidity and mortality
- Muscle weakness, as measured by reduced grip strength in the lowest 20% at baseline, adjusted for gender and body mass index (BMI)
- Physical slowness, based on measured time to walk a distance of 15 feet, at usual pace
- Poor endurance, as indicated by self-reported exhaustion
- Low physical activity, as scored using a standardized assessment questionnaire

Sleep problems

Sleep problems have different expression and high prevalence in the older adult. In the Well-being Singapore Elderly Study, a cross-sectional, epidemiologic survey conducted among Singapore residents aged 60 years and above (n = 2565), the older adults reported at least 1 sleep problem, with the overall prevalence of 13.7% (n = 341).[3]

In this study, the sleep problems reported consisted of sleep interruption at night, having difficulty falling asleep, and early awakening. The patient conditions were characterized by chronic physical conditions, depression, and low physical activity.

Sleep problems can affect quality of life and can contribute to falls, injuries, and other health problems. Having trouble sleeping at night or feeling sleepy during the day may be indicative of sleep problems.

Bladder control problems

Bladder control problems, or urinary incontinence, in older persons, is highly prevalent, increasing in older patients as they progress in years, and is reported more by woman. Bladder incontinence may be caused by conditions such as age-related changes in the lower urinary tract, urinary tract infection, and conditions not directly related to the genitourinary system, such as diabetes, cancer, stroke, cognitive impairment, and mobility impairment. Urinary incontinence also can lead to problems such as falls, depression, and isolation.

Delirium
Delirium is a sudden change in mental function in an older person, a serious situation that requires immediate attention of a health care professional. Delirium is common at the emergency room or during hospital admissions. It usually occurs in 2 forms: a hyperactive form, in which patients are agitated, have increased arousal, or are very vigilant, or a hypoactive form in which patients are lethargic, sleepy, move less than usual, and have little awareness of their surroundings.

Dementia
Dementia is a memory problem significant enough to affect one's ability to carry out usual tasks. Although the most common cause is Alzheimer disease, there are many other types.

Falls
Falls are a leading cause of serious injury in older people. There are many risk factors for falling, including safety hazards in the home, medication side effects, walking and vision problems, dizziness, arthritis, weakness, and malnutrition. Like other geriatric syndromes, falls usually have more than 1 cause.

Osteoporosis
Osteoporosis is a condition that makes the bones of older adults more fragile and easy to break. Women 65 and older, and men over age 70, should get a bone mass density (BMD) test. Increased calcium and vitamin D intake, strength training exercises, and weight-bearing exercises such as walking are important for keeping healthy bones.

Weight loss
Weight loss is a very common problem in older adults. Weight loss can be caused by the diminished sense of taste that comes with aging, or it can be a suggestion of an underlying serious medical problem. No matter the cause, weight loss can lead to other problems, such as weakness, falls, and bone disorders.

CLINICAL PHARMACOLOGY
Definition

Clinical pharmacology is defined as the use of pharmacology therapeutic agents in the prevention, treatment, and control of disease in people.

Geriatric patients are a subset of older people with multiple comorbidities having significant functional implications. Geriatric patients have impaired homeostasis and wide interindividual variability. Comprehensive geriatric assessment captures the complexity of the problems that characterize frail older patients and can be used to guide management, including prescribing. Prescribing for geriatric patients requires an understanding of the efficacy of the medication in frail older people, assessment of the risk of adverse drug events, discussion of the harm: benefit ratio with the patient, a decision about the dose regime and careful monitoring of the patient's response.[4]

Prescribing for older adults by its nature has several challenges. The physiologic changes in the process of normal aging, genetics, added environment influences, diseases, and other factors as the ones related to the use of drugs, chemical, and toxic products make each patient unique for evaluation and continuous management.

Compared with younger adults, elderly adults have lower physiologic reserve, and are placed in a condition of fragility when suffering from an acute or chronic health disorder.

Clinically there is a decrease in muscle mass and strength, bone density, ability to perform exercises, respiratory function, thirst, and nutrition as well as the immunologic capacity. As a result, patients may be exposed to prolonged periods of bed rest and immobility are also very sensitive to unexpected climatic fluctuations.

There are many treatments available for these conditions that can help maintain independence and improve quantity and quality of life.

Pharmacokinetics

Pharmacokinetics is how the body manages the drugs from the moment they are swallowed or the way that they were administered, to the point of elimination. There are different processes or transformations and changes that alter the effect of medications in the body, resulting in a prolonged impact in elderly patients. Parenteral loading doses need to be adjusted for body weight, but volume of distribution has little changes.

These processes include: absorption, distribution, metabolism, and elimination. All of them can vary with age, gender, through innate or inherited changes, environmental effect, disease, or medication use.

AGE-RELATED CHANGES IN PHARMACOKINETICS AND THE ELDERLY
Absorption

Age-related gastrointestinal tract and skin changes seem to be of minor clinical significance for medication usage. Most drugs require passive diffusion and no change in bioavailability, and drugs that require active transport may have decreased bioavailability. Decreased first-pass effect on hepatic metabolism will increase bioavailability.

Distribution

Important age-related changes include

- Decrease in lean body mass and total body weight
- Increased percentage of body fat
- Increase in volume of distribution for lipophilic drugs, such as sedatives that penetrate the central nervous system (CNS)
- Protein-binding changes are of modest significance for most drugs, especially at steady-state

Metabolism

Although liver function tests are unchanged with age, there is some overall decline in metabolic capacity. Decreased liver mass and hepatic blood flow are the most significant changes. Metabolism can affect drugs such as lidocaine, propranolol, and morphine.

Excretion

Age-related decreased renal blood flow and glomerular filtration rate (GFR) are well-established. Metabolism can affect drugs such as lidocaine, propanolol and morphine. Serum creatinine may not be a good predictor of renal function. There may be marked renal impairment.

PHARMACODYNAMICS

Pharmacodynamics is how the drug acts over the body or the physiologic effect of the drugs over end–organ function. Factors are those influencing actual sensitivity to a particular concentration of the drug at the tissue level. These factors determine the degree of therapeutic response and whether an adverse effect will occur.

For example, digoxin is cleared by the kidney and generally given to geriatric patients at half the usual adult dose in order to compensate for age-related diminution in (GFR); this is a pharmacokinetic change. The presence of disease in the target organ (heart) could result in an enhanced effect of digoxin, even in appropriate doses leading to a toxic arrhythmia; this is a pharmacodynamic change.

RISK OF POLYPHARMACY IN THE GERIATRIC PATIENT
Polypharmacy

Polypharmacy is the use of 4 or more medications or the administration of more medication than clinically indicated. The risk of polypharmacy occurs with prescribed drugs, over the counter (OTC) drugs, herbal substances, and also treatment or diagnostic procedures. The impact of polypharmacy on the elderly population is significant. It is associated with poor adherence with treatment regimen, drug-drug interactions, medication errors, and adverse drug reactions. The consequence may result in medical conditions and injuries, including falls, hip fractures, confusion, delirium, and emergency room visits and hospitalization.

Important factors that lead to polypharmacy in the elderly are conditioned by interactions between physiologic reserves, functional, and cognitive status; and formal or informal support system availability, resulting in a situation of added vulnerability. Polypharmacy occurs in combination therapy or polytherapy used in a single disease condition or when involved in multiple comorbidities.

Another significant problem of polypharmacy is in terms of both direct and indirect medication costs, that may produce drug-related morbidity with impact in the personal economy of the patient and in the corresponding health system.

Several circumstances may increase the risk of polypharmacy; one is known as prescribing cascades. In this circumstance, the effects of a drug are misdiagnosed as symptoms of another problem, resulting in further prescriptions and further adverse effects.

There are other situations in which the patient is overwhelmed by a complicated medical regimen, making medication errors more likely. This can lead to toxicity or lower therapeutic effect, involving or leading to polypharmacy. To optimize the desired results of the drug and minimize adverse effects, there are some recommendations.

Patient at Risk Evidence-Based Strategies

One essential strategy is to identify, stratify, and target individual patients at higher risk of polypharmacy and adverse drug events (ADEs). These patient characteristics can be classified into 3 groups:

1. Demographic (increasing age, white race, female gender, higher levels of education)
2. Health status (general poor health, cardiovascular disease, hypertension, asthma, diabetes)
3. Access to health care (increased number of health care visits, multiple providers, type of insurance)

INTERVENING TO REDUCE POLYPHARMACY AND SIMPLIFIED MEDICATION REGIMEN

First determine if the problem exists, identify the degree and magnitude[5]:

- Obtain a geriatric drug history about the medications the patient is taking with dosage, duration, and indication of each; include pills, creams, OTC drugs and other nonprescription vitamins, supplements, and herbal substances

- ○ Assess why the patient is using them now, his or her understanding about effectiveness and knowledge of adverse reaction and side effects
- Reconciliation of patient list with the office list of medications

HOW TO SIMPLIFY A MEDICATION REGIMEN

If an adverse event or reaction occurs, do not add a drug, take 1 away. Discontinue all drugs considered unnecessary or of uncertain therapeutic efficacy. Identify the over-treated patient.

INAPPROPRIATE MEDICATION USE

There are some drug categories of concern in the elderly that pose risks for this age group, including analgesics, anticoagulants, antihypertensive drugs, antiparkinsonian drugs, diuretics, hypoglycemic drugs, and psychoactive drugs. They are classified as potentially inappropriate medications (PIMs) and are prescribed and used preponderantly in clinical practice for the most vulnerable of patients-the older adults.

TOOLS TO HELP DECREASE POTENTIALLY INAPPROPRIATE DRUG USE

The American Geriatrics Society (AGS) Beers Criteria for Potentially Inappropriate Medication Use in Older Adults (2015) update is applicable to all older adults with the exclusion of those in palliative and hospice care. Rigorous application of the criteria by health professionals, consumers, payors, and health systems should lead to closer monitoring of drug use in older adults. It is the most commonly used tool.[6]

The STOPP criteria or Screening Tool Of Older Persons' Potentially Inappropriate Prescriptions are comprised of 65 clinical criteria, more common avoidable practices some of them overlapping with Beers criteria.[6,7]

The START criteria or Screening Tool to Alert Doctors to Right Treatments are used in conjunction with STOPP criteria to identify correct treatments for elderly. They are composed of 22 criteria.[6,7]

MEDICATION ERRORS

A medication error refers to oversights (of commission or omission) at any step along the pathway that begins when a clinician prescribes a medication and ends when the patient actually receives the medication.[8]

This pathway consists of 4 steps: prescribing, transcribing, dispensing, and administration.

The first 2 steps comprise the more susceptible to commit error within the all process.

Prescribing

Avoid unnecessary medications following conservative prescribing principle.

Use computerized provider order entry (CPOE) to eliminate hand writing errors, combining with clinical decision support systems and medication reconciliation.

Medication reconciliation is a formal process of obtaining and verifying a complete and accurate list of each patient's current medicines. During this process, the clinician matches the medicines the patient should be prescribed to those they are actually prescribed.

Transcribing and Dispensing

Use CPOE for transcribing. For dispensing, use a medication dispensing process under supervision of a clinical pharmacist.

Administration

Adhere to the "Five Right" rule of medication safety: administering the right medication, in the right dose, at the right time, by the right route, to the right patient. Use the barcode in medication administration to ensure the medication is given to the correct patient. Minimize interruption to allow the nurse to administer medication safely. Use an infusion pump for intravenous infusions. Patients should be educated, and medication levels should be revised.

Although most errors likely occur at the prescribing and transcribing stages, medication administration errors are also common in inpatient and outpatient settings. Preventing medication errors requires specific steps to ensure safety at each stage of the pathway.

Judicious prescribing

Judicious prescribing[9] is a prerequisite for safe and appropriate medication use. Based on evidence from studies demonstrating problems with widely prescribed medications as was previously identified as PIMs, here is offered a series of principles as a prescription for more cautious and conservative prescribing.

These principles urge clinicians to

1. Think beyond drugs (consider nondrug therapy, treatable underlying causes, and prevention)
2. Practice more strategic prescribing (defer nonurgent drug treatment, avoid unwarranted drug switching, be circumspect about unproven drug uses, and start treatment with only 1 new drug at a time)
3. Maintain heightened vigilance regarding adverse effects (suspect drug reactions, be aware of withdrawal syndromes and educate patients to anticipate reactions)
4. Exercise caution and skepticism regarding new drugs (seek out unbiased information, wait until drugs have sufficient time on the market, be skeptical about surrogate rather than true clinical outcomes, avoid stretching indications; avoid seduction by elegant molecular pharmacology, beware of selective drug trial reporting)
5. Work with patients for a shared agenda (do not automatically accede to drug requests, consider nonadherence before adding drugs to regimen, avoid restarting previously unsuccessful drug treatment, discontinue treatment with unneeded medications, and respect patients' reservations about drugs)
6. Consider long-term, broader impacts (weigh long-term outcomes and recognize marginal benefits of new drugs).

REFERENCES

1. Dong X, Milholand B, Vijg J. Evidence for a limit to human lifespan. Nature 2016; 538(7624):257–9. Available at: www.nature.com/nature/journal/v538/n7624/abs/nature19793.html.
2. Ortman JM, Velkoff VA, Hogan H. An aging nation: the older population in the United States. Population estimates and projections. Current population reports. Mortality: Driver of Trends in the Older Population. US Census Bureau. 2014. p. 25–1140.
3. Sagayadevan V, Abdin E, Shafie SB, et al. Prevalence and correlates of sleep problems among elderly Singaporeans. Psychogeriatrics 2017;17(1):43–51.

Wiley Online Library. Available at: http://onlinelibrary.wiley.com/doi/10.1111/psyg. 12190/full.
4. Hilmer SN, McLachlan AJ, Le Couteur DG. Clinical pharmacology in the geriatric patient. Fundam Clin Pharmacol 2007;21(3):217–30.
5. Pretorius RW, Gataric G, Swedlund SK, et al. Reducing the risk of adverse drug events in older adults. Am Fam Physician 2013;87(5):331–6.
6. By the American Geriatrics Society 2015 Beers Criteria Update Expert Panel. American Geriatrics Society 2015 updated Beers criteria for potentially inappropriate medication use in older adults. J Am Geriatr Soc 2015;63(11):2227–46.
7. O'Mahony D, O'Sullivan D, Byrne S, et al. STOPP/START criteria for potentially inappropriate prescribing in older people: version 2. Age Ageing 2015;44(2): 213–8.
8. Medication errors | AHRQ Patient Safety Network. 2015. Available at: https://psnet. ahrq.gov/primers/primer/23/medication-errors. Accessed July 25, 2017.
9. Schiff GD, Galanter WL, Duhig J, et al. Principles of conservative prescribing. Arch Intern Med 2011;171(16):1433–40.

Nutritional Needs of the Older Adult

Melissa Bernstein, PhD, RD, LD, FAND

KEYWORDS

- Anorexia of aging • Sarcopenic obesity • Food desert • Food insecurity
- Artificial nutrition and hydration

KEY POINTS

- Ensuring adequate nutritional intake for all older adults is an essential factor in promoting health and well-being, and maintaining functional independence.
- Adequate nutritional intake can prevent comorbidities such as increased susceptibility to acute and chronic illness, impaired immune function, and malnutrition.
- The ability to consume the appropriate quality and quantity of foods is influenced by food accessibility, availability, acceptability (preference), preparation, and the eating process itself.
- Age-related changes in nutrient digestion, absorption, and metabolism contribute to alterations in dietary requirements for macronutrients, vitamins, and minerals, underscoring the need for nutrient-dense foods.
- The role of nutrition in health promotion and disease prevention is evolving with strategies designed to meet the needs of the aging individual.

INTRODUCTION

Nutrition is well-recognized as one of the major determinants of successful aging and a key means for avoiding age-related physical and mental deterioration. Nutritional inadequacy can interfere with health and the ability to remain independent, and lead to complications such as increased burdens of poor health, polypharmacy, reduced socialization, and limited functional ability. This article provides an overview of some of the requirements, challenges, and services to promote optimal nutritional intake for older adults.

DIETARY GUIDANCE FOR OLDER ADULTS

The goal of nutrition recommendations in the aging population is one of disease management and also of health protection so that individuals can live long and enjoy good

Disclosures: M. Bernstein receives a portion of author royalties from Jones and Bartlett Learning in association with the publication of Nutrition, Discovering Nutrition, Nutrition for Older Adults and Nutrition Across Life Stages.
Department of Nutrition, Chicago Medical School, Rosalind Franklin University of Medicine and Science, 3333 Green Bay Road, North Chicago, IL 60064, USA
E-mail address: melissa.bernstein@rosalindfranklin.edu

Phys Med Rehabil Clin N Am 28 (2017) 747–766
http://dx.doi.org/10.1016/j.pmr.2017.06.008
1047-9651/17/© 2017 Elsevier Inc. All rights reserved.

health. Older adults often have numerous medical conditions that require a change in food or nutrient intake. Maintaining a nutrient-dense diet is essential to promoting health and preventing nutrition-related complications that could contribute to declining health, functional dependency, and frailty. Although older adults are discussed as a group, the actual nutritional needs and challenges of individuals are as unique as the older adults themselves.

DIETARY GUIDELINES FOR AMERICANS AND MyPlate

Lifelong dietary patterns affect the likelihood of age-related chronic disease. Regardless of age, eating healthful foods and limiting poor food choices should be a priority. For adults of every age, low-fat dairy, lean meats, adequate fiber, whole grains, fruits, and vegetables should be emphasized. *Trans* fats, sodium, sugar, and excess calories should be minimized. The *2015-2020 Dietary Guidelines for Americans* (the *Dietary Guidelines*) and MyPlate offer dietary guidance for whole foods and food groups rather than individual nutrients.[1,2] For older adults, eating nutritious food without overconsuming calories can be a challenge in the face of functional dependence, frailty, and illness. Tufts University's MyPlate for Older Adults highlights the unique dietary needs of adults older than 70 years by additionally emphasizing fluid intake, and nutrient-dense food choices such as protein-rich foods, vegetables, fruits, whole grains, healthy oils, and low-fat dairy choices.[3] The topic area of "older adults" is new for *Healthy People 2020* and was developed in response to the rapidly aging American population. The aim of the older adult initiative is to "improve the health, function, and quality of life of older adults."[4]

As an older individual's health declines, the need to individualize nutritional recommendations is of significant importance, especially in the presence of multiple disease conditions. Older adults at risk of malnutrition or undesirable weight loss should have their diets liberalized if possible to promote adequate food and nutrient intake. Strict restrictions such as a low-salt diet, for example, may actually decrease food intake because of lack of flavor.

THE DIETARY REFERENCE INTAKES

For most older adults, aging is a continuum of deteriorating health and functionality leading to increased disability and dependency, which in turn further influence an individual's nutritional needs. Although chronologic age is used as a cutoff for the Dietary Reference Intakes (which include the age categories 51–70 years, and >70 years), actual nutrient requirements may be wide-ranging in the older adult population. Selected nutrients of concern in older adults are discussed in **Table 1**.

NUTRIENT RECOMMENDATIONS AND REQUIREMENTS
Energy

Energy intake and energy requirements commonly decrease with advancing age. This causes a challenge for many older individuals because, although they require fewer calories to maintain their weight, nutrient needs stay the same and, in some cases, increase.[5,6] Meeting nutrient recommendations while simultaneously maintaining a healthful weight is fundamental to dietary guidance for older adults. Lower energy requirements result from decreased energy expenditure, losses in lean body mass, and reduced physical activity. Older adults who do not reduce their caloric intake to balance a decrease in energy expenditure are at risk for overweight, obesity, and

Table 1
Nutrient concerns in older adults

Nutrient	Considerations for the Older Adult
Energy	Requirements for energy to maintain a healthy body weight usually decline for older adults. Nutrient-dense foods help to meet nutritional requirements and maintenance of a healthy body weight.
Protein	High-quality protein evenly distributed throughout the day.
Fluids	Sufficient fluids must be provided in efforts to prevent dehydration. Adequate fluids sustain homeostasis in the body and aid in moving nutrients to cells, metabolizing medications, and eliminating waste products.
Fiber	Fiber is important for gastrointestinal health, improves lipoprotein levels, reduces risk factors for coronary heart disease, and aids in weight management and the maintenance of normal blood glucose levels. Consuming too much fiber can cause gastrointestinal distress and too little fiber can lead to constipation.
Calcium	Calcium is essential in promoting healthy bones and teeth. Calcium also has an important role in blood clotting, muscle contraction, and nerve transmission.
Vitamin D	Vitamin D is essential in promoting bone health. Vitamin D has a well-established function in bone metabolism, calcium homeostasis, and the prevention of osteoporosis. Higher levels of vitamin D have been found to be associated with a reduction in cancer risk. Vitamin D has also been found to exert a protective effect against cardiovascular disease, arthritis, multiple sclerosis, and diabetes mellitus.
Zinc	Zinc is a functional component of many enzymes and proteins and is involved in the regulation of gene expression. Zinc deficiency can contribute to conditions common in the older adult, such as loss of appetite, hair loss, delayed wound healing, skin abnormalities, impaired taste, and depression.
Folate	Adequate folate functions with vitamins B_6 and B_{12} in the metabolism of methionine and homocysteine. Deficiency can cause megaloblastic anemia and hyperhomocysteinemia. High consumption of folic acid can mask a serious vitamin B_{12} deficiency.
Vitamin B_{12}	Vitamin B_{12} is a coenzyme in nucleic acid metabolism. Deficiency causes megaloblastic anemia. Older adults may have suboptimal levels of vitamin B_{12} owing to inadequate diet or poor absorption resulting from a lack of intrinsic factor or atrophic gastritis. Vitamin B_{12} deficiency can lead to changes in mental status, peripheral neuropathy, balance disturbances, and hyperhomocysteinemia.
Iron	Iron is a structural component of hemoglobin. Iron deficiency leads to microcytic hypochromic anemia. Iron deficiency in older adults is frequently caused by a gastrointestinal bleed, poor nutrition intake, and medication side effects.
Carotenoids	Carotenoids with vitamin A activity such as lutein and zeaxanthin are found in the macula of the eye and may help to prevent the onset and progression of age-related macular degeneration. Carotenoids with antioxidant activity can help reduce the risk of cataracts.

Data from Institute of Medicine, Food and Nutrition Board. Dietary reference intakes: the essential guide to nutrient requirements. Washington, DC: National Academies Press; 2006. Available at: https://fnic.nal.usda.gov/sites/fnic.nal.usda.gov/files/uploads/DRIEssentialGuideNutReq.pdf. Accessed September 27, 2016; and Institute of Medicine, Food and Nutrition Board. Dietary reference intake: calcium and vitamin D. Washington, DC: National Academies Press; 2011. Available at: https://fnic.nal.usda.gov/sites/fnic.nal.usda.gov/files/uploads/FullReport.pdf. Accessed September 27, 2016.

associated complications, metabolic consequences, and comorbidities. Therefore, the importance of older adults making nutritious foods choices is paramount.

Carbohydrates and Fiber

For health promotion and disease prevention, the *Dietary Guidelines* recommend that carbohydrate requirements be met with nutritious whole grains, fruits, and vegetables, which are also high in fiber. Limiting processed foods and sugar intake is also emphasized. Foods high in added sugar are low in nutrients, high in calories, and crowd out more nutritious options.

Consumption of fiber-rich foods helps with the management of body weight and diabetes mellitus, and reduces the risk of cardiovascular disease and various types of cancer. Foods that contain high amounts of insoluble fiber increase fecal bulk and decrease transit time in the colon, helping to lower the incidence of constipation and formation of diverticula, conditions common in older adults. Fiber-rich foods delay gastric emptying into the small intestine, resulting in the sensation of fullness, which although beneficial for weight loss, can be a problem for frail and underweight older adults struggling to consume adequate calories and meet nutritional requirements.

Fiber consumption is consistently lower than recommended levels for older adults.[7] Recommendations range from 25 to 35 g/d, with the adequate intake for total fiber set at 30 g/d for men and 21 g/d for women older than the age of 51 (based on 14 g fiber per 1000 kcal).[8] Choosing a variety of fiber-rich foods such as fruits, vegetables, legumes, whole grains, and high-fiber breakfast cereals is the best way to increase fiber consumption. When including foods high in fiber, it is particularly important that older adults meet fluid recommendations to prevent constipation and fecal impaction.

Fat

For healthy older adults, keeping fat and carbohydrate intake within recommended ranges helps to lower the risk for chronic disease. Older adults should choose dietary fats in similar distributions to those recommended for younger adults, including aiming for less than 10% of total calories from fats and limiting *trans* fats to less than 0.5% of total calories. Dietary fat provides a necessary source of the essential fatty acids linoleic acid (*n*-6), an omega-6 fatty acid, and linolenic acid (*n*-3), an omega-3 fatty acid. In older adults, essential fatty acids may have the potential to prevent and reduce comorbidities; are associated with lower total mortality, particularly from heart disease; and may have beneficial effects on inflammation markers.[9–13] Omega-3 fatty acids in particular may have substantial benefits for reducing the risk of cognitive decline in older people, potentially treating age-related memory disorders, and also for maintaining muscle performance and immune function.[9] Additionally, fat is a valuable source of concentrated energy for frail and underweight older adults.

Protein

Eating enough high-quality dietary protein may be challenging for older adults, especially for those with reduced appetite, functional and social limitations, and economic hardship. Dietary protein requirement for this diverse population continues to be a topic of scientific investigation. The current Recommended Dietary Allowance (RDA) is 56 g/d for males and 46 g/d for females, or 0.80 g/kg body weight per day of protein based on nitrogen balance studies.[8] Some experts propose that the RDA for protein may not be adequate to meet the metabolic and physiologic needs even as a minimum level for older adults.[14] Moderate increases in protein intake above 0.80 g/kg/d may contribute to enhanced muscle protein metabolism, and provide a mechanism for reducing progressive muscle loss that commonly accompanies aging.[15] A protein intake of 1.2 g/kg body weight per day, either by improving diet or by adding protein supplements, has been suggested to help older adults maintain and regain lean body mass and function.[16] In general, experts recommend that protein intake range from 1.0 to 1.5 g/kg daily, with the higher end of this range needed to meet additional demands of physiologic stress such as for those with impaired absorption and hypercatabolic conditions, such as infections, decubitus ulcers, and cancer, but only for persons without any overt renal dysfunction.[17] To meet this recommendation, an even distribution of protein-rich foods throughout the day is suggested for older adults, translating to approximately 30 g of high-quality protein 3 times a day.[18,19] Increased frailty, sarcopenia, skin fragility, impaired wound healing, and impaired immune function are all consequences of reduced body proteins.[15]

Fluids

Water is an essential nutrient that requires special attention for older adults. Water constitutes approximately 10% to 15% less of an older adult's body weight than in younger adults.[20] Endocrine and renal changes, hemodynamic factors, environmental factors, decreased sensation of thirst, medication use, and voluntary restriction can reduce intake and make older adults vulnerable to fluid imbalance. The adequate intake for total water is set at 2.7 and 3.7 L daily for women and men ages 51 and older, respectively, an amount intended to prevent dehydration.[21] Water intake should correspond with calorie intake with 35 mL/kg of body weight per day.[22–24]

Fluid intake may be influenced by many factors in older adults, such as those listed in **Box 1**. Dehydration can be life threatening and has been called the most common fluid and electrolyte disturbance in older adults.[25] Medications require adequate fluid for proper metabolism, so poor fluid status and dehydration can alter medication function and effectiveness. Dehydration is common among older people living in long-term care facilities.[26] A wide range of interventions can reduce its prevalence, but more work is this area is needed and will likely require the coordination of an interprofessional team of providers, including caregiver staff, health care policymakers, and researchers.[27,28]

MICRONUTRIENTS: VITAMINS AND MINERALS

Age-related changes in nutrient absorption or metabolism can contribute to higher dietary requirements for many vitamins and minerals. Recommended intakes of vitamins and minerals for older adults attempt to take into consideration the variability among this age group by offering recommendations for those ages 51 to 70 years, and for those ages 70 and older.[29]

B Vitamins

The vitamins B_{12}, B_6, and folate are of special interest in the older population. An estimated 6% of adults aged 60 or older are vitamin B_{12} deficient, and approximately 20% have borderline low levels.[30] In institutionalized elderly residents, the prevalence of vitamin B_{12} deficiency can reach almost 35%.[31] Vitamin B_{12} deficiency is characterized by neurologic abnormalities, including cognitive decline, peripheral neuropathy, decreased muscle strength, and functional disability.[32] Decreased gastric acid, lack of intrinsic factor, atrophic gastritis with accompanying small bowel bacterial overgrowth, and certain medications interfere with normal vitamin B_{12} absorption in many older adults.[33] As a result of these gastric changes, it can be easier for older adults to absorb synthetic vitamin B_{12} from supplements and fortified foods than

---

Box 1
Factors that can influence fluid intake in older adults

- Changes in mental status, cognitive ability, memory loss, and depression.
- Diminished thirst sensations owing to changes in the hypothalamus.
- Incontinence.
- Inability to get and drink liquids owing to physical limitations, poor strength, risk of falling, or functional declines.
- Not wanting to drink because of dysphagia and choking or dislike of thickened liquids as part of the dysphagia diet.
- Restricting fluids because of early satiety.
- History of not consuming enough fluids.
- Drinking results in dysgeusia, or a bad taste.
- Too fatigued to drink enough fluids.
- Gastric upset with drinking certain beverages.
- Lack of taste or appeal of beverages.
- Fear of drinking, owing to dementia or agitation, or fear of the person offering the beverage.
- Side effects of medications that interfere with fluid intake, alterations in urinary or gastrointestinal function, nausea, or confusion.
- Attitudes and beliefs regarding drinking.

Adapted from Heuberger RA. Geriatric Nutrition Table 15.4 factors that can influence fluid intake in older adults. In: Bernstein MA, McMahon K, editors. Nutrition across life stages. Burlington (MA): Jones and Bartlett Learning; 2018; and Begg DP. Disturbances of thirst and fluid balance associated with aging. Physiol Behav 2017;178:28–34; with permission.

---

the B_{12} that is naturally found in foods. A daily consumption of 2.4 mg of vitamin B_{12} is suggested for all adults 51 years and older.[29]

Vitamins B_{12}, B_6, and folate act together to metabolize homocysteine, a nonessential sulfur-containing amino acid. The Third National Health and Nutrition Examination Survey found that approximately 14% of older persons had hyperhomocysteinemia.[34] Hyperhomocysteinemia is an independent risk factor for cardiovascular diseases and mortality, and plays an important role in atherosclerosis, neurodegenerative, and cognitive impairment, as well as in dementia, diabetes mellitus, decreased skeletal health, gastrointestinal disorders, and immune responses.[35,36] Homocysteine levels can be lowered with supplemental vitamins B_6, vitamin B_{12}, and folate. Folic acid supplementation in excess of recommended levels can mask a vitamin B_{12} deficiency.

Calcium and Vitamin D

Calcium and vitamin D are well-known for their primary roles in bone health. Calcium has other essential roles in the blood and extracellular fluid and in vasodilation and vasocontraction, muscle contraction, blood clotting, and nerve transmission.[6] Vitamin D has a direct effect on skeletal muscle formation by promoting protein synthesis and increases intestinal calcium uptake. Vitamin D has also been found to exert a protective effect against cardiovascular disease, arthritis, multiple sclerosis, cancer, and diabetes mellitus.[37] Older adults deficient in vitamin D are more likely to have limitations in mobility and physical performance and function, whereas adequate vitamin D has been found to reduce the risk of falling by more than 20%.[38,39] Low levels of vitamin D have recently been associated with symptoms of depression in older adults, possibly through a biologic role in the brain affecting memory, motor control, and social behaviors.[40] Sufficient vitamin D and protein are needed as part of nutritional strategies to increase muscle mass in older adults with sarcopenia.[41]

Calcium and vitamin D intakes of older adults are frequently lower than recommended. For people aged 51 to 70 years, the RDA for calcium is 1200 mg/d for women and 1000 mg/d for men. The calcium RDA for people 70 years of age and older is 1200 mg/d.[6] It can be challenging for older adults to consume the recommended amount of calcium and vitamin D from food alone. Low-fat dairy products are good sources of calcium, vitamin D, and protein and are low in calories and fat, making them a worthy food choice for older adults; however, calcium and vitamin D supplementation may also be needed in this population.[42]

Vitamin D insufficiency is common in the older population because of lower dietary intake, and decreased skin synthesis and renal production of vitamin D. Older adults staying indoors have limited sunlight exposure and those with lactose intolerance avoid dairy products. The National Academy of Medicine (formerly the Institute of Medicine) has vitamin D requirements set at 600 IU for adults ages 51 to 70 years and 800 IU for adults older than 70 years.[43] Research suggests adults need at least 1000 to 2000 IU/d of vitamin D to achieve adequate serum levels.[44]

Sodium

Advice to follow a healthy eating pattern that is low in sodium is part of the *Dietary Guidelines* because even modest reductions in sodium intake are associated with substantial health benefits.[1] More than 70% of the sodium in the American diet is present at high levels in food before it is even served.[45] Almost 50% of the sodium in the US diet comes from mixed dishes (such as burgers, sandwiches, rice, pasta, grain dishes, pizza, meat, poultry, seafood dishes, and soups), foods commonly consumed by older adults. High-protein foods, grains, vegetables, snacks, sweets, dairy, and condiments also contribute sodium.[1,46] The Tolerable Upper Intake Level for sodium is 2300 mg (1 teaspoon) for adults ages 51 and older.[21] However, more than 85% of adults older than 51 years of age have a usual daily intake of 3293 mg.[47]

There is strong evidence of a dose–response effect of sodium reduction on blood pressure and that reducing dietary sodium prevents cardiovascular disease.[48,49] Older adults with hypertension can follow the Dietary Approaches to Stop Hypertension dietary plan, which is lower in sodium than the typical American diet and reduces risk factors for cardiovascular disease. The Dietary Approaches to Stop Hypertension plan is high in vegetables, fruits, low-fat dairy products, whole grains, poultry, fish, beans, and nuts; it is low in sweets, sugar-sweetened beverages, and red meats. The Dietary Approaches to Stop Hypertension diet is also low in saturated fats and rich in potassium, calcium, magnesium, dietary fiber, and protein.[50] Frequent monitoring of older adults prescribed a low-sodium diet is recommended because, although the sodium restriction has been shown to lower blood pressure, it may contribute to a bland diet, decrease food intake, and negatively affect nutritional status.[51]

Iron

Iron deficiency is not a common condition in older adults because average dietary iron intake for older adults is usually above the RDA of 8 mg/d for men and women ages 51 and older and iron losses owing to menstruation in women ceases with menopause.[52] Iron deficiency, however, can occur with poor intake over a long period of time, gastrointestinal bleeding, or from prolonged malabsorption or other medical conditions.[52] Low iron levels can lead to anemia and symptoms such as decreased energy, episodes of syncope, pale skin, irregular heartbeat, cold extremities, and headaches. Reduced meat consumption associated with taste changes, medication use, economics, and poor dentition can contribute to low iron intake. Important dietary sources of iron for older adults are those that are well-absorbed, such as beef, fish, pork, tofu, legumes, and fortified breakfast cereals. Older adults with iron deficiency anemia will likely require iron supplementation.

Zinc

Although zinc deficiency is rare, the average zinc intake for older adults tends to be below the RDA of 8 mg/d for adult women and 11 mg/d for adult men.[52] There is no consistent evidence that aging affects zinc absorption or that requirements are greater in older adults. If a deficiency exists, zinc supplementation could benefit immune function in older adults.[52] Zinc supplementation for the prevention or treatment of age-related macular degeneration (AMD) remains questionable, but may slow the progression of AMD to an advanced stage.[53] Results from the AREDS2 study found no significant progression of AMD with the low-zinc AREDS formula when compared with the high-zinc formula.[54] Stress, particularly in hospitalized older adults, may increase the risk for low zinc levels and impaired immune function. Multivitamin supplementation is recommended for patients with pressure injuries, or with diagnosed or suspected zinc deficiencies. Zinc supplementation does not seem to improve wound healing.[55] Excess zinc may actually inhibit healing, affect immune function, alter the absorption of other minerals, and may lower high-density lipoprotein cholesterol levels. Supplementation should be supervised medically.

Antioxidants

Aging results in increased oxidative stress, which increases further with most chronic diseases. An eating pattern that contains a substantial amount of antioxidants is associated with the maintenance of physiologic functions in older adults and a lower prevalence of degenerative diseases. Antioxidants may protect against brain impairment that may result in Alzheimer disease and other cognitive deteriorations common in aging.[56] Specifically, vitamins E and C, and vitamin A carotenoids have been identified as nutrients involved in reducing disease rates through several protective mechanisms. Vitamin E functions primarily as a chain-breaking antioxidant, maintaining cell integrity by preventing lipid peroxidation, and it plays a role in immune function and the blood clotting process. Good sources of vitamin E include vegetable oil, nuts, seeds, whole grains, and dark green leafy vegetables. Vitamin C is a potential preventive agent against cognitive impairment; serves a vital role in collagen synthesis, wound healing, and immune function; and facilitates iron absorption.[57–59] Vitamin C is found mainly in fruits and vegetables. Carotenoids have antioxidant properties and protect against free radicals that result in tissue damage and increased risk of age-related diseases. Carotenoids provide protection against various cancers, AMD, dementia, cardiovascular disease, and arthritis.[58] When the physiologic demand for antioxidants is high, low blood levels may occur, which could affect disease progression and the aging process.[60]

Diets high in antioxidant-rich foods such as fruits and vegetables have been associated with a lower incidence of cardiovascular disease, AMD, and cancer. Higher mortality, however, has been associated with high-dose nutrient supplements, suggesting a threshold level for these nutrients and toxic effects can occur at higher supplement intakes.[61] Older adults should therefore aim to boost their food sources of antioxidants and use dietary supplements only when necessary, with medical supervision.

Alcohol

Alcohol intake in moderation has been shown to have some beneficial health effects in adults. However, older persons are far more likely to experience negative outcomes owing to changes in the body's processing of alcohol. Older adults, particularly those with medical conditions and those taking multiple medications, are at increased risk of adverse events related to alcohol including falls, accidents, and drug–ethanol interactions, as well as complications from existing disease states and comorbid conditions. Psychological conditions common in this age group such as depression, anxiety, bereavement, social isolation, and life changes (eg, retirement) may precipitate late-onset heavy drinking or alcohol abuse.[17]

From a nutritional perspective, alcohol is a significant source of empty calories, providing 7 calories per gram. High quantities of alcohol intake can displace necessary nutrients, decrease appetite, alter taste perception, and interfere with the absorption, use, and homeostasis of nutrients in older adults already having difficulty meeting nutritional recommendations and at risk of malnutrition.[62,63]

NUTRITIONAL AND DIETARY SUPPLEMENTS

The majority (if not all) of the nutrients an older adult consumes should come from food rather than supplements, to the extent possible.[33] Many older adults, however, find it difficult to eat enough nutrient-dense foods to meet their needs, so nutrient supplementation may be indicated to maintain health and body weight. Numerous dietary supplements and nutritional products are marketed to older adults using targeted advertising.[64] More than one-half of older adults report using complementary and alternative medicine and more than a one-third, including almost 25% of those aged 85 years and older, take some type of herbal product or dietary supplement.[65] Older adults use dietary supplements to prevent illness, for overall wellness, to reduce pain and treat painful conditions, to treat specific health conditions, and to supplement conventional medical treatments. Yet more than two-thirds of adults do not discuss their supplement use with a health care provider, often because they do not consider herbs or dietary supplements medications.[65] Health care professionals working with older adults should ask about the use of complementary medicine and dietary supplement use (including herbal supplements, carotenoids, and phytochemicals) and monitor for polypharmacy, potentially harmful interactions, and side effects.

BODY SYSTEM CHANGES AND NUTRITIONAL STATUS IN OLDER ADULTS

Eighty-five percent of noninstitutionalized older adults have at least 1 chronic health condition that could be improved with proper nutrition.[66] Efforts to consume a nutritious diet can be influenced by health status and factors that may occur naturally with aging or as a result of illness and interfere with and older adult's ability to meet their nutritional needs, especially when calorie needs are reduced. Age-related changes in the body may influence how a disease manifests and progresses, as well as its severity (**Table 2**). Most disability of old age is associated with age-dependent conditions that have nutritional implications, such as coronary heart disease, adult-onset diabetes, and Alzheimer's disease, which are ultimately the main causes of death in persons older than the age of 65.[66]

Table 2
Nutritional implications of age-related changes in body systems

Body System	Impact on Nutrition	Health-Related Consequence
Decreased total energy expenditure	Decreased energy requirements Increased importance of nutrient-dense food choices	Increased risk of obesity
Decreased muscle mass and strength	Functional impairment could limit food access Decreased need for energy Increased need for high-quality protein	Changes in body composition favor an increased risk for sarcopenia, frailty, and functional dependency
Reduced skin synthesis of vitamin D (cholecalciferol)	Increased requirement for vitamin D and calcium	Decreased bone density and skeletal mass Increased risk for bone fractures and osteoporosis
Decreased kidney function	Reduced ability to concentrate urine contributes to increased fluid needs	Increased risk for dehydration Alterations in drug metabolism
Decreased immune function	Increased needs for high-quality proteins, antioxidants, vitamin B_6, vitamin E, and zinc	Increased susceptibility to illness and disease
Gastrointestinal changes	Age-related changes in gastrointestinal function, specifically, nutrient digestion and absorption, can influence nutrient status and requirements	Malnutrition can result for inadequate nutrient digestion and absorption or other gastrointestinal complications
Oral cavity	The first signs of micronutrient deficiencies and malnutrition often appear in the oral tissues	Chronic diseases and medications in older adults can lead to complications in the oral cavity that result in pain, tooth loss, xerostomia, and problems with chewing and swallowing, changes in taste and smell which contribute to poor appetite and impaired ability to eat and drink
Esophageal function	Reduced food and nutrient intake	Dysphagia is common in older adults with neurodegenerative diseases such as dementia or stroke and psychiatric diseases
Gastric function GERD, atrophic gastritis, and increased gastric pH	Increased requirements for folate, calcium, vitamin K, vitamin B_{12}, and iron	Increased risk for pernicious anemia and vitamin B_{12} deficiency
Slowed gastric motility	Increased need for fluids and fiber	Increased risk for constipation

Adapted from Bernstein MA. Older adult nutrition. In: Bernstein MA, McMahon K, editors. Nutrition across life stages. Burlington (MA): Jones and Bartlett Learning; 2018. p. 454–5; with permission.

Body Composition

Changes in body composition in older adults favor a loss of lean body mass and increases in body fat, which contribute to poor health, functional impairment, and disease comorbidities. These changes interfere with the ability to maintain independence in daily activities and result in increased frailty, declining physical functioning, and worsening health.[33] Sarcopenia may affect up to 33% of community-dwelling older adults, with a higher prevalence in frail elders in long-term care and acute care settings, and an estimated cost of $18.5 billion.[67,68] Sarcopenia is an independent risk factor for numerous adverse outcomes, difficulties with activities of daily living and instrumental activities of daily living, osteoporosis, falls, hospital duration of stay and readmission, and death.[67] Some nutrition interventions being investigated include nutritional supplements, the amount and timing of dietary protein, essential amino acids, β-hydroxyl β-methylbutyrate, vitamin D, dietary acid–base load, fatty acids, and antioxidants.[67,69]

Overweight and Obesity

More than 30% of adults age 65 and older are obese from poor food choices, primarily the consumption of a low-quality diet with too many calories and physical inactivity.[70] Obesity contributes to increased morbidity, reduced quality of life, and increased risk for a significant number of chronic diseases in older adults.[71] Energy-restricted, high-protein diets benefit health profiles, including improvements in fasting glucose and lipids of obese older adults at risk for chronic disease when combined with resistance training.[72] Although a concern in terms of comorbidities and managing disease symptoms and risk factors, the presence of obesity can have a protective effect against unintentional and involuntary weight loss in older adults.

Sarcopenic Obesity

The simultaneous occurrence of sarcopenia and obesity, termed sarcopenic obesity, is detrimental to physical functioning and the health of older adults and contributes to worsening of health status.[73] Physical exercise, specifically progressive resistance strength training, is the most effective intervention to prevent and reverse sarcopenia.[74] Optimizing nutritional intake, in particular adequate high-quality protein and antioxidants, is important. Interventions that combine exercise with dietary strategies can prevent and manage sarcopenia in older adults.[75]

Weight Loss and Malnutrition

As many as one-half of noninstitutionalized older adults may be malnourished.[66] Malnourished older adults are more prone to infections and diseases, their injuries take longer to heal, surgery is riskier, and their hospital stays are longer and more expensive. Restrictive medical diets can become unpalatable and unenjoyable, thus worsening food intake and nutritional status, and should be liberalized to the extent possible to minimize undesirable weight loss.[76] Some older adults will experience weight loss owing to anorexia of aging (age-associated changes in appetite regulation and lack of hunger). Anorexia of aging can result from a combination of physiologic, social, and pathologic conditions and may lead to protein–energy malnutrition and weight loss.[77] Dietary interventions for older adults should maximize treatment, respect aging body systems, preserve quality of life, and support overall well-being.

Other Body Systems

Older individuals have an increased susceptibility to gastrointestinal complications, hypertension, cardiovascular disease, and deteriorating neurologic functioning.

Age-related changes and diseases affect the functioning of the renal, immune, skeletal, nervous, and endocrine systems. Careful diagnosis of any underlying diseases and conditions and appropriate medical nutrition therapy are crucial to the successful nutritional management of older adults.

FACTORS THAT AFFECT DIET AND FOOD INTAKE IN OLDER ADULTS

Nutrition impacts how a person will age; in turn, the process of aging affects nutritional needs. Numerous factors affect adequate food intake, making the task of maximizing nutrition in older adults complicated. Each adult arrives at old age with different nutritional requirements built on lifelong eating behaviors influenced by physiologic, behavioral, social, environmental, and psychological factors. Food provides more than just nourishment for older adults; it also contributes to a sense of security and gives meaning and structure to the day. Mealtime is often an opportunity for socialization and psychological well-being. **Table 3** lists factors affecting the food intake and nutritional status of older adults.

HEALTH, MEDICAL, AND PHYSICAL FACTORS THAT INFLUENCE DIET

Arthritis, cardiovascular disease, diabetes, cancer, obesity, osteoporosis, gastroesophageal reflux disease, food intolerances, alcoholism, poor oral health, pressure injuries, anorexia of aging, malnutrition, constipation, and dehydration can result from chronic dietary inadequacies and require dietary modifications as part of their treatment.[78] Medications can cause side effects that affect food intake, lower appetite, influence the absorption or metabolism of nutrients, or lead to changes in taste

Table 3
Summary of factors that affect food intake and nutritional status of older adults

Medical/Physiologic Alterations	Physical Changes	Social, Cultural, and Economic Factors
Chronic illness and conditions	Changes in physical endurance, strength and balance	Living arrangement
Acute illnesses		Access to transportation
Polypharmacy: prescription and over-the-counter medication use including dietary supplements and complementary practices.	Functional status and mobility	Proximity to major grocery store
	Physical abilities and limitations	Socioeconomic status and finances
Changes in nutrient absorption and digestion	Ability to self-feed	Social support of friends, family, and caregivers
Changes in mental status, memory loss, and depression	Ability to obtain and prepare food	Lifelong dietary habits and food preferences, spiritual, ethnic practices, and religious beliefs
Problems with oral health, such as difficulty chewing, and swallowing		Education and literacy
Changes in taste perception and olfactory ability		
Changes in vision		
Anorexia of aging		
Health status necessitating a modified diet or MNT		

Adapted from Bernstein MA. Older adult nutrition. In: Bernstein MA, McMahon K, editors. Nutrition across life stages. Burlington (MA): Jones and Bartlett Learning; 2018; with permission.

and smell that make food unappealing. Illness and depression can reduce an older adult's willingness to cook and eat meals. Changes in vision, oral health, and dentition, as well as declines in taste and smell, are often overlooked, but can affect an older person's ability to prepare and enjoy meals. Independence and functional status directly impact food intake and nutritional status. Physical limitations can make the simple tasks of shopping and cooking overwhelming, leading to progressive worsening of nutritional status, which further impairs health and well-being.

ENVIRONMENTAL, SOCIAL, AND CULTURAL FACTORS THAT AFFECT DIET

Psychological factors that have a strong influence on an individual's nutritional well-being include food security, education, finances, literacy, language, and cultural beliefs. Ethnic, cultural, and long-standing food-related behaviors have a significant effect on food choice and preparation methods. Older individuals are more likely than younger individuals to maintain habitual and cultural food choices, which necessitates dietary guidance that is considerate of food preferences and access to culturally acceptable foods.

Too many older adults face food insecurity, the risk of not having adequate money to buy food. Food-insecure individuals might adopt problematic coping strategies, such as limiting meal sizes or spending money on medications instead of food. For community-dwelling older adults living in food deserts (geographic areas, especially rural or impoverished urban locations, lacking accessible supermarkets or grocery stores), dependency on transportation and limited finances affect their ability to purchase wholesome foods. Financially challenged older adults who rely on convenience stores have higher average food costs, further reducing their food purchasing power.[79]

PROMOTING NUTRITION AND HEALTHY LIFESTYLES FOR OLDER ADULTS

Food not only is critical to one's physiologic well-being, but also contributes to quality of life. Many older adults require specialized nutrition services to maintain their independence and health. Enabling older adults to stay at home and in their communities versus in institutional care helps to preserve higher quality of life, reduce long-term health care costs, and maintain their independence and ties to family and friends.[80,81]

NUTRITION PROGRAMS FOR OLDER ADULTS

The aim of the home and community-based long-term care system is to promote health through an array of services, including nutrition programs, that help to maintain the quality of life and independence of older adults and prevent or delay institutionalization. Participation in food and nutrition programs can improve dietary quality and health indicators for older adults. Federal food and nutrition assistance programs are a critical source of nutrition support for many older adults. The Administration on Aging, a branch of the US Department of Health and Human Services, is responsible for administering nutrition services to America's older adults. The Administration on Aging was established to carry out the Older Americans Act of 1965, which "promotes the well-being of older individuals by providing services and programs designed to help them live independently in their homes and communities."[82] The Older Americans Act Nutrition program is the largest national food and nutrition program specifically designed to serve older adults. There are a number of programs intended to fight hunger that service older adults including Congregate Nutrition Services and Home-Delivered Nutrition Services supported by the Administration on

Aging and the Nutrition Services Incentive Program, the Federal Supplemental Nutrition Assistance Program (formerly the Food Stamp Program), Commodity and Supplemental Foods, the Emergency Food Assistance Program, the Child and Adult Care Food Program, and the Senior Farmers' Market Nutrition Program.[83–85] Nutrition programs aimed at promoting health in older adults should be integrated into the overall health care plan.

PHYSICAL ACTIVITY

Physical activity and exercise have consistently been linked with diseases and conditions that have significant nutritional implications in older adults. Regular physical activity is associated with lower mortality rates; chronic disease prevention, reduction, and management; and improved mental and cognitive capability, depressive states, psychological health, independence, balance, bone strength, muscular strength, and overall quality of life across the life span.[86,87] Physical activity and age-appropriate exercise interventions have the potential to reduce disease risk factors, increase and preserve skeletal muscle mass, improve functional status and quality of life, stimulate appetite, and prevent disability at any age.

CLINICAL AND END-OF-LIFE NUTRITION AND HYDRATION CONSIDERATIONS

At the end of life, older adults are vulnerable to poor decision making, abuse, and neglect. Appropriate and compassionate end-of-life care, including attention to nutrition and hydration, should be made while the older adult is able to communicate their wishes soundly. It is common to have an interprofessional heath care team involved with end of life care decision making of frail geriatric patients.

There are several methods for feeding a person at the end of life. The expression "food first" continues to apply into old age if the person is able to eat. When a person is unable to eat enough to maintain body weight, artificial nutrition and hydration may be used to supplement or replace oral intake. If the gastrointestinal tract is still well-functioning, a nasogastric tube can be used. Feeding this way still uses the stomach, but is quick and ensures that enough nutrients are consumed. A percutaneous endoscopic gastrostomy tube can be placed laparoscopically and a supplemental nutrition formula poured through the tube directly into the lumen of the stomach. As a last resort, total parenteral nutrition can be used for feeding and hydrating a geriatric patient.

The recent popularity of "right to die" and "voluntary refusal of food and fluids" movements demonstrates the heightened awareness of end-of-life nutrition and hydration issues.[88] Providing food and fluids gives the appearance of "doing something" to care for a family's loved one. Some patients, however, may voluntarily refuse food and water referred to as "voluntary stopping of eating and drinking." When a person is near death, they often naturally do not want to eat or drink, and there is evidence to suggest that feeding and hydrating someone who is close to death may cause them to be more uncomfortable.[17] There is a legal and ethical obligation to honor the rights of an individual when making decisions on providing, withdrawing, or withholding food and water, as long as they are competent to make those decisions.

SUMMARY

Good nutrition is a critical component of healthy aging. The maintenance of good health for the growing population of older adults requires approaches that recognize multiple levels of influence on the individual—medical, social, cultural, environmental, organizational, and personal factors. It can be difficult for older adults to meet their nutritional needs because of their increased requirements for some nutrients, lower energy needs, and numerous health and lifestyle barriers to adequate food intake. Age-related changes in health influence digestion, absorption, and metabolism of foods and nutrients, translating to changes in nutritional requirements. There are significant challenges to healthy eating for older adults, especially those with chronic conditions, physical limitations, and financial constraints, as well as those who reside in different settings. The decreased food intake, sedentary lifestyle, and reduced energy expenditure commonly seen in older adults places them at risk for malnutrition, especially protein and micronutrient deficiencies. Persistent, chronic conditions create additional challenges for older adults to carry out their activities of daily living, including food-related tasks. Older adults should be encouraged to consume a variety of nutrient-dense foods, and supplementation should be considered when dietary intake is inadequate. Delivering nutrition services and programs is vital to making a positive impact in the lives of older adults. Health care providers have opportunities to develop care plans that can help older adults to promote and maintain their health. More attention, resources, and nutrition expertise are needed to meet the food and nutrition requirements of vulnerable older adults so that they can live independently with a good quality of life.

ACKNOWLEDGMENTS

The author acknowledges the assistance of Nancy Munoz, DCN, MHA, RDN, FAND, Robin B. Dahm, RDN, LDN, and Eva Kaminski Shaw, BA, in reviewing this article.

REFERENCES

1. US Department of Health and Human Services and US Department of Agriculture. 2015 – 2020 Dietary Guidelines for Americans. 8th edition. 2015. Available at: http://health.gov/dietaryguidelines/2015/guidelines/. Accessed March 13, 2017.
2. US Department of Agriculture. USDA Choose MyPlate.Gov. Available at: https://www.choosemyplate.gov/dietary-guidelines. Accessed March 13, 2017.
3. Tufts University nutrition scientists provide updated MyPlate for Older Adults. Tufts University website. Available at: http://now.tufts.edu/news-releases/tufts-university-nutrition-scientists-provide-updated-myplate-older-adults. Accessed March 13, 2017.
4. Office of Disease Prevention and Health Promotion. Healthy People 2020 topics and objectives: older adults. HealthyPeople.gov website. Available at: http://www.healthypeople.gov/2020/topicsobjectives2020/overview.aspx?topicid=31. Accessed March 13, 2017.
5. Otten JJ, Pitzi Hellwig J, Meyers LD, editors. Institute of Medicine. Dietary reference intakes: the essential guide to nutrient requirements. Washington, DC: National Academies Press; 2006. Available at: https://fnic.nal.usda.gov/sites/fnic.nal.usda.gov/files/uploads/DRIEssentialGuideNutReq.pdf. Accessed March 13, 2017.
6. Institute of Medicine, Food and Nutrition Board. Dietary reference intakes: calcium and vitamin D. Washington, DC: National Academies Press; 2011. Available at: https://fnic.nal.usda.gov/sites/fnic.nal.usda.gov/files/uploads/FullReport.pdf. Accessed March 13, 2017.
7. Hoy MK, Goldman JD. Fiber intake of the U.S. population: What We Eat in America, NHANES 2009–2010. Food Surveys Research Group Dietary Data Brief No. 12. September 2014.

8. Institute of Medicine, Food and Nutrition Board. Dietary reference intakes for energy, carbohydrate, fiber, fat, fatty acids, cholesterol, protein and amino acids (macronutrients). Washington, DC: National Academies Press; 2005.

9. Molfino A, Gioia G, Rossi Fanelli F, et al. The role for dietary omega-3 fatty acids supplementation in older adults. Nutrients 2014;6(10):4058–73.

10. Mozaffarian D, Lemaitre RN, King IB, et al. Plasma phospholipid long-chain ω-3 fatty acids and total and cause-specific mortality in older adults: a cohort study. Ann Intern Med 2013;158(7):515–25.

11. Wilk JB, Tsai MY, Hanson NQ, et al. Plasma and dietary omega-3 fatty acids, fish intake, and heart failure risk in the Physicians' Health Study. Am J Clin Nutr 2012; 96(4):882–8.

12. Johnson GH, Fritsche K. Effect of dietary linoleic acid on markers of inflammation in healthy persons: a systematic review of randomized controlled trials. J Acad Nutr Diet 2012;112(7):1029–41.

13. Chiuve SE, Rimm EB, Sandhu RK, et al. Dietary fat quality and risk of sudden cardiac death in women. Am J Clin Nutr 2012;96(3):498–507.

14. Volpi E, Campbell WW, Dwyer JT, et al. Is the optimal level of protein intake for older adults greater than the Recommended Dietary Allowance? J Gerontol A Biol Sci Med Sci 2013;68(6):677–81.

15. Paddon-Jones D, Rasmussen BB. Dietary protein recommendations and the prevention of sarcopenia. Curr Opin Clin Nutr Metab Care 2009;12(1):86–90.

16. Bauer J, Biolo G, Cederholm T, et al. Evidence-based recommendations for optimal dietary protein intake in older people: a position paper from the PROT-AGE Study Group. J Am Med Dir Assoc 2013;14:542–59.

17. Heuberger RA. Geriatric nutrition. In: Bernstein MA, McMahon K, editors. Nutrition across life stages. Burlington (MA): Jones and Bartlett Learning; 2018. p. 493–531.

18. Cardon-Thomas DK, Riviere T, Tieges Z, et al. Dietary protein in older adults: adequate daily intake but potential for improved distribution. Nutrients 2017; 9(3):184.

19. Mamerow MM, Mettler JA, English KL, et al. Dietary protein distribution positively influences 24-h muscle protein synthesis in healthy adults. J Nutr 2014;144: 876–80.

20. Popkin BM, D'Anci KE, Rosenburg IH. Water, hydration, and health. Nutr Rev 2010;68(8):439–58.

21. Institute of Medicine, Food and Nutrition Board. Dietary reference intakes for water, potassium, sodium, chloride, and sulfate. Washington, DC: National Academies Press; 2004.

22. Schnelle J, Leung F, Rao S, et al. A controlled trial of an intervention to improve urinary and fecal incontinence and constipation. J Am Geriatr Soc 2010;58(8): 1504–11.

23. Godfrey H, Cloete J, Dymond E, et al. An exploration of the hydration care of older people. Int J Nurs Stud 2012;49(10):1200–11.

24. Hoope L, Bunn D, Jimi F, et al. Water loss and dehydration in aging. Mech Ageing Dev 2014;136(137):50–8.

25. Weinberg AD, Minaker KL. Dehydration: evaluation and management in older adults. JAMA 1995;274:1552–6.

26. Hooper L, Bunn DK, Downing A, et al. Which frail older people are dehydrated? The UK DRIE study. J Gerontol A Biol Sci Med Sci 2016;71(10):1341–7.

27. Bunn D, Jimoh F, Wilsher SH, et al. Increasing fluid intake and reducing dehydration risk in older people living in long-term care: a systematic review. J Am Med Dir Assoc 2015;16(2):101–13.

28. Keller H, Beck AM, Namasivayam A. International-Dining in nursing home Experts (I-DINE) consortium improving food and fluid intake for older adults living in long-term care: a research agenda. J Am Med Dir Assoc 2015;16(2):93–100.

29. Institute of Medicine. Dietary reference intakes: vitamins. Institute of Medicine. Available at: http://www.nationalacademies.org/hmd/~/media/Files/Activity%20Files/Nutrition/DRI-Tables/2_%20RDA%20and%20AI%20Values_Vitamin%20and%20Elements.pdf?la=en. Accessed March 13, 2017.

30. Allen LH. How common is vitamin B-12 deficiency? Am J Clin Nutr 2009;89(2): 693S–6S.

31. Wong CW, Ip CY, Leung CP, et al. Vitamin B12 deficiency in the institutionalized elderly: a regional study. Exp Gerontol 2015;69:221–5.

32. Oberlin BS, Tangney CC, Gustashaw KAR, et al. Vitamin B12 deficiency in relation to functional disabilities. Nutrients 2013;5(11):4462–75.

33. Bernstein M, Munoz N, Academy of Nutrition and Dietetics. Position of the Academy of Nutrition and Dietetics: food and nutrition for older adults: promoting health and wellness. J Acad Nutr Diet 2012;112:1255–77.

34. Pfeiffer CM, Caudill SP, Gunter EW, et al. Analysis of factors influencing the comparison of homocysteine values between the Third National Health and Nutrition Examination Survey (NHANES) and NHANES 1999. J Nutr 2000;130:2850–4.

35. Ganguly P, Alam SF. Role of homocysteine in the development of cardiovascular disease. Nutr J 2015;14:6.

36. Schalinske KL, Smazal AL. Homocysteine imbalance: a pathological marker. Adv Nutr 2012;3(6):755–62.

37. National Institutes of Health, Office of Dietary Supplements. Health information: vitamin D fact sheet for health professionals. National Institutes of Health, Office of Dietary Supplements; 2016. Available at: http://ods.od.nih.gov/factsheets/VitaminD-HealthProfessional/. Accessed March 13, 2017.

38. Sohl E, van Schoor NM, de Jongh RT, et al. Vitamin D status is associated with functional limitations and functional decline in older individuals. J Clin Endocrinol Metab 2013;98(9):E1483–90.

39. Houston DK, Neiberg RH, Tooze JA, et al. Low 25-hydroxyvitamin D predicts the onset of mobility limitation and disability in community-dwelling older adults: the Health ABC Study. J Gerontol A Biol Sci Med Sci 2013;68(2):181–7.

40. Milaneschi Y, Hoogendijk W, Lips P, et al. The association between low vitamin D and depressive disorders. Mol Psychiatry 2014;19(4):444–51.

41. Verlaan S, Maier AB, Bauer JM, et al. Sufficient levels of 25-hydroxyvitamin D and protein intake required to increase muscle mass in sarcopenic older adults - The PROVIDE study. Clin Nutr 2017. [Epub ahead of print].

42. Sahni S, Mangano KM, Kiel DP, et al. Dairy intake is protective against bone loss in older vitamin d supplement users: the Framingham Study. J Nutr 2017. http://dx.doi.org/10.3945/jn.116.240390.

43. Institute of Medicine of the National Academies. Dietary reference intakes for calcium and vitamin D. 2010. Available at: http://www.nationalacademies.org/hmd/Reports/2010/Dietary-Reference-Intakes-for-Calcium-and-Vitamin-D/DRI-Values.aspx. Accessed March 13, 2017.

44. Boucher BJ. The problems of vitamin D insufficiency in older people. Aging Dis 2012;3(4):313–29.

45. Frieden TR. Sodium reduction – saving lives by putting choice into consumers' hands. JAMA 2016;316(6):579–80.
46. Hoy MK, Goldman JD, Murayi T, et al. Sodium Intake of the U.S. Population: What We Eat In America, NHANES 2007–2008. Food Surveys Research Group Dietary Data Brief No. 8. 2011. Available at: http://ars usda gov/Services/docs htm?docid=19476. Accessed March 13, 2017.
47. Centers for Disease Control and Prevention. Prevalence of excess sodium intake in the United States – NHANES, 2009-2012. MMRW Morb Mortal Wkly Rep 2016; 64(52):1393–7. Available at: https://www.cdc.gov/mmwr/preview/mmwrhtml/mm6452a1.htm?s_cid=mm6452a1_w. Accessed March 14, 2017.
48. Cogswell ME, Mugavero K, Bowman BA, et al. Dietary sodium and cardiovascular disease risk—measurement matters. N Engl J Med 2016;375:580–6.
49. Mozaffarian D, Fahimi S, Singh GM, et al, Global Burden of Diseases Nutrition and Chronic Diseases Expert Group. Global sodium consumption and death from cardiovascular causes. N Engl J Med 2014;371(7):624–34.
50. National Heart, Lung, and Blood Institute. Description of the DASH eating plan. National Heart, Lung, and Blood Institute; 2015. Available at: http://www.nhlbi.nih.gov/health/health-topics/topics/dash. Accessed March 13, 2017.
51. Gunn JP, Barron JL, Bowman BA, et al. Sodium reduction is a public health priority: reflections on the Institute of Medicine's report, sodium intake in populations: assessment of evidence. Am J Hypertens 2013;26(10):1178–80.
52. Institute of Medicine. Dietary reference intakes for vitamin A, vitamin K, arsenic, boron, chromium, copper, iodine, iron, manganese, molybdenum, nickel, silicon, vanadium, and zinc. Washington, DC: National Academies Press; 2001.
53. Vishwanathan R, Chung M, Johnson EJ. A systematic review on zinc for the prevention and treatment of age-related macular degeneration. Invest Ophthalmol Vis Sci 2013;54(6):3985–98.
54. Gorusupudi A, Nelson K, Bernstein PS. The age-related eye disease study: Micronutrients in the treatment of macular degeneration. Adv Nutr 2017;8:40–53.
55. Posthauer ME, Banks M, Dorner B, et al. The role of nutrition for pressure ulcer management: national pressure ulcer advisory panel, European Pressure Ulcer Advisory Panel, and Pan Pacific Pressure Injury Alliance white paper. Adv Skin Wound Care 2015;28(4):175–88.
56. Devore E, Kang J, Stampfer M, et al. Total antioxidant capacity of diet in relation to cognitive function. Am J Clin Nutr 2010;92:1157–64.
57. National Institutes of Health, Office of Dietary Supplements. Health information: vitamin C fact sheet for health professionals. National Institutes of Health, Office of Dietary Supplements; 2016. Available at: https://ods.od.nih.gov/factsheets/VitaminC-HealthProfessional/. Accessed March 13, 2017.
58. National Institutes of Health, Office of Dietary Supplements. Health information: vitamin A fact sheet for health professionals. National Institutes of Health, Office of Dietary Supplements; 2016. Available at: https://ods.od.nih.gov/factsheets/VitaminA-HealthProfessional/. Accessed March 13, 2017.
59. National Institutes of Health, Office of Dietary Supplements. Health information: vitamin E fact sheet for health professionals. National Institutes of Health, Office of Dietary Supplements; 2016. Available at: https://ods.od.nih.gov/factsheets/VitaminE-HealthProfessional/. Accessed March 13, 2017.
60. Saffel-Shrier S. Vitamin requirements of the older adult. In: Bernstein M, Munoz N, editors. Nutrition for the older adult. 2nd edition. Burlington (MA): Jones & Bartlett Learning; 2016. p. 73–90.

61. Goyal A, Terry MD, Siegel AB. Serum antioxidant nutrients, vitamin A, and mortality in US adults. Cancer Epidemiol Biomarkers Prev 2013;22(12):2202–11.
62. Heuberger RA. Alcohol and the older adult: a comprehensive review. J Nutr Elder 2009;28(4):203–35.
63. Kuerbia A, Sacco P, Blazer D, et al. Substance abuse among older adults. Clin Geriatr Med 2014;30(3):629–54.
64. Montalto C, Bhargva V, Hong SG. Use of complementary and alternative medicines by older adults. Evid Based Complement Alternat Med 2006;11(17):27–46.
65. National Center for Complementary and Integrative Health. Complementary and alternative medicine: what people aged 50 and older discuss with their health care providers. National Center for Complementary and Integrative Health; 2015. Available at: https://nccih.nih.gov/research/statistics/2010. Accessed March 14, 2017.
66. Chernoff R. Geriatric nutrition: the health professional's handbook. 4th edition. Burlington (MA): Jones & Bartlett Learning; 2013.
67. Cruz-Jentoft AJ, Landi F, Schneider SM, et al. Prevalence of and interventions for sarcopenia in ageing adults: a systematic review. Report of the International Sarcopenia Initiative (EWGSOP and IWGS). Age Ageing 2014;43(6):748–59.
68. Janssen I, Shepard DS, Katzmarzyk PT, et al. The healthcare costs of sarcopenia in the United States. J Am Geriatr Soc 2004;52(1):80–5.
69. Hickson M. Conference on 'Nutrition and age-related muscle loss, sarcopenia and cachexia' Symposium 3: Nutrition for prevention and interventions for sarcopenia and cachexia. Nutritional interventions in sarcopenia: a critical review. Proc Nutr Soc 2015;74:378–86.
70. Federal Interagency Forum on Aging-Related Statistics. Older Americans 2010: key indicators of well-being. Washington, DC: U.S. Government Printing Office; 2010. Available at: http://agingstats.gov/docs/PastReports/2010/OA2010.pdf. Accessed March 13, 2017.
71. Kyrgiou M, Kalliala I, Markozannes G, et al. Adiposity and cancer at major anatomical sites: umbrella review of the literature. BMJ 2017;356:j477.
72. Amamou T, Normandin E, Pouliot J, et al. Effect of a high-protein energy-restricted diet combined with resistance training on metabolic profile in older individuals with metabolic impairments. J Nutr Health Aging 2017;21(1):67–74.
73. Houston DK, Nicklas BJ, Zizza CA. Weighty concerns: the growing prevalence of obesity among older adults. J Am Diet Assoc 2009;109(11):1886–95.
74. Beaudart C, Dawson A, Shaw SC, et al, IOF-ESCEO Sarcopenia Working Group. Nutrition and physical activity in the prevention and treatment of sarcopenia: systematic review. Osteoporos Int 2017. http://dx.doi.org/10.1007/s00198-017-3980-9.
75. Denison HJ, Cooper C, Sayer AA, et al. Prevention and optimal management of sarcopenia: a review of combined exercise and nutrition interventions to improve muscle outcomes in older people. Clin Interv Aging 2015;10:859–69.
76. Dorner B, Friedrich EK, Posthauer ME, American Dietetic Association. Position of the American Dietetic Association: individualized nutrition approaches for older adults in health care communities. J Am Diet Assoc 2010;110:1549–53.
77. Wysokińsk A, Sobów T, Kłoszewska I, et al. Mechanisms of the anorexia of aging-a review. Age 2015;37:81.
78. Bernstein MA. Older adult nutrition. In: Bernstein MA, McMahon K, editors. Nutrition across life stages. Burlington (MA): Jones and Bartlett Learning; 2018. p. 451–534.

79. Sharkey JR, Dean WR, Nalty C. Convenience stores and the marketing of foods and beverages through product assortment. Am J Prev Med 2012;43(3S2): S109–15.

80. Kamp BJ, Wellman NS, Russell C, Position of the American Dietetic Association, American Society for Nutrition, Society for Nutrition Education. Position of the American Dietetic Association, American Society for Nutrition, and Society for Nutrition Education: food and nutrition programs for community-residing older adults. J Am Diet Assoc 2010;110:463–72.

81. Office of Disease Prevention and Health Promotion. Home and community-based services 1915(c). Medicaid.gov website. Available at: http://www.medicaid.gov/Medicaid-CHIP-Program-Information/By-Topics/Long-Term-Services-and-Supports/Home-and-Community-Based-Services/Home-and-Community-Based-Services-1915-c.html. Accessed March 14, 2017.

82. US Department of Health and Human Services (USDHHS). Administration for community living. Administration on Aging (AOA). Available at: https://aoa.acl.gov/. Accessed March 14, 2017.

83. USDA Programs and Services. Available at: https://www.fns.usda.gov/programs-and-services. Accessed March 14, 2017.

84. Nutrition.gov Food Assistance Programs. Nutrition programs for seniors. Available at: https://www.nutrition.gov/food-assistance-programs/nutrition-programs-seniors. Accessed March 14, 2017.

85. US Department of Health and Human Services (USDHHS). Administration for Community Living. Administration on Aging (AOA). Nutrition Services (OAA Title IIIC). Available at: https://aoa.acl.gov/AoA_Programs/HPW/Nutrition_Services/index.aspx Accessed March 14, 2017.

86. Sun F, Norma IJ, White AE. Physical activity in older people: a systematic review. BMC Public Health 2013;13:449.

87. World Health Organization. Global Strategy on Diet, Physical Activity and Health: global recommendations on physical activity for health. World Health Organization. Available at: http://www.who.int/dietphysicalactivity/factsheet_recommendations/en/. Accessed March 14, 2017.

88. O'Sullivan Maillet J, Baird Schwartz D, Posthauer ME, Academy of Nutrition and Dietetics. Position of the academy of nutrition and dietetics: ethical and legal issues in feeding and hydration. J Acad Nutr Diet 2013;113:828–33.

The Competitive Senior Athlete

David A. Soto-Quijano, MD

KEYWORDS

- Older athletes • Sports medicine • Master athletes • Chronic diseases
- Cardiovascular diseases • Diabetes mellitus • Medication complications
- Dehydration

KEY POINTS

- As the population ages, more individuals older than the age of 65 will have the opportunity to participate in a variety of fitness activities and competitive sports.
- Even though there may be a possible cause and effect relationship between some sports and osteoarthritis, there is evidence that exercise reduces pain and enhances physical function of the affected joints.
- The risk of sudden cardiac death increases with physical activity; however, there is a consensus that health benefits of regular physical exercise far outweigh the acutely increased risk of this condition.
- Older athletes should ingest fluids before and during sports competitions, because there is an increased risk of dehydration in that age group.
- The use of medications and dietary supplements is common among older athletes. Clinicians should be aware about the possible effects of medications on sports performance.

INTRODUCTION

In the year 2017 the National Senior Games Association will be celebrating 30 years of their first competition. In that initial event, which was held in St. Louis, Missouri, close to 2500 competitors older than the age of 50 participated in 15 sports. In the year 2015, the number of participants grew to almost 10,000 athletes.[1] With the well-discussed aging of the population more individuals older than the age of 65 will have the opportunity to participate in a variety of fitness activities and competitive sports. Clinicians should be prepared to treat older athletes and help them to continue their active lifestyles. This article discusses some of the unique medical challenges that this population presents.

Disclosure Statement: The author has nothing to disclose.
Physical Medicine and Rehabilitation Residency Program, VA Caribbean Healthcare System, 10 Casia Street (117), San Juan, PR 00921, USA
E-mail address: David.soto-quijano@va.gov

Phys Med Rehabil Clin N Am 28 (2017) 767–776
http://dx.doi.org/10.1016/j.pmr.2017.06.009
1047-9651/17/© 2017 Elsevier Inc. All rights reserved.

First we need to define older athletes. Other terms that have been used to describe this group include master athletes, mature athletes, and aged athletes. An athlete is defined as a person who commits to their sport or activity at least five times a week with the activity level achieved being more than what is recommended for general health benefits, resulting in the heart beating significantly faster and shortness of breath that makes talking difficult.[2] Another simpler and more inclusive description of an athlete is a person who participates in an organized team or individual sport that requires regular competition against others as a central component, places a high premium on excellence and achievement, and requires some form of systematic (and usually intense) training.[3]

What constitutes a senior athlete will depend on the sport or the events. The National Senior Games includes athletes that are older than 50 years. World Masters Athletic includes women and men of age 35 and older and divides them into 5-year groups up to age 100. To play in the Senior Professional Golf Association tour the athlete must be older than 50 years. The International Tennis Federation divides their older players into three divisions. The young seniors age categories range from 35 to 45 for men and women, the seniors range from 50 to 60, and the super-seniors range from 65 to 85 for men and 60 to 80 for women.[4] The American College of Sports Medicine/American Heart Association physical activity and public health recommendations for older adults suggest that, in most cases, "old age" guidelines apply to individuals aged 65 years or older, although they can also be relevant for adults aged 50 to 64 years with clinically significant chronic conditions or functional limitations.[5]

When treating older athletes, one should contemplate each patient's goal. Some patients compete sporadically just for fun, but some others want to achieve a high level of skill that allows them to participate in organized competitions. Also consider if the patient is an experienced athlete who has been participating in their sports for most of their life or a newcomer that started practicing sports during their adult years. For some competitors their athletic achievements are a source of great pride and an important part of their lives, so it is imperative for them to heal fast and get back to competition as soon as possible. As health care professionals we understand that returning to sports is equally important to all patients regardless of their goals, because it is an important part of a healthy lifestyle.[5]

There is evidence that physical activity significantly reduces the risk of many medical problems and that master athletes have a lower risk of chronic diseases than their sedentary counterparts.[6] However, advancing age is associated with an increased risk of for chronic diseases.[5] Some of the conditions that older athletes may suffer and important considerations that are helpful to manage this important group are discussed next.

THE OLDER ATHLETE AND DIABETES

It is estimated that there are 11.2 million people 65 years and older who suffer from diabetes mellitus in the United States.[7] Studies have shown that the decline in glucose tolerance and insulin sensitivity that is commonly seen with aging and that may lead to this condition is prevented in some individuals with regular exercises.[8] Master athletes with an average age of 60 years were found with normal glucose tolerance and lower plasma insulin levels (fasting and after glucose ingestion) when compared with older, untrained men. The master athletes' blood glucose and insulin levels were found as low as in young athletes.[9] A group of master runners and triathletes with an average age of 63.5 years showed enhanced insulin sensitivity and a lower waist-to-hip ratio when compared with age- and body fat–matched sedentary individuals.[10] Furthermore, lifestyle interventions including regular exercise can reduce the risk of diabetes even in subjects who have already been found with impaired glucose tolerance.[11]

Just like in the younger population, athletes with type 2 diabetes mellitus are at a higher risk of hypoglycemia and should monitor their glucose levels closely during competitions. It is recommended to log glucose levels before, during, and after exercising to determine the best way to use nutritional or pharmacologic treatments to achieve a healthy glycemic control throughout their athletic activity.[12] Also consider that regular exercise may cause the athlete to lose weight and become more insulin sensitive. Once again, the pharmacologic and nutritional regiment needs to be re-evaluated closely to avoid periods of hypoglycemia or hyperglycemia. The use of medical alert identifications should be encouraged during competitions if permitted, in case the athlete develops a complication during the event and requires medical care.

Possible diabetes complications should also be considered. There is no evidence that exercise and physical activity can have an adverse effect on vision or the progression of nonproliferative diabetic retinopathy or macular edema. However, in the presence of proliferative or severe nonproliferative diabetic retinopathy, vigorous aerobic or resistance exercise may be contraindicated because of the risk of triggering vitreous hemorrhage or retinal detachment.[13] Peripheral neuropathy may affect the patient's performance and increase the risk of injury, but once again there is no published evidence. In severe cases, patients are at risk of developing Charcot joint, so non-weight-bearing sports should be encouraged. Physical activity can acutely increase urinary protein excretion, so caution should be taken in patients with microalbuminuria and nephropathy. The magnitude of this increase is in proportion to the acute increase in blood pressure, so it is recommended that people with diabetic kidney disease perform only light or moderate exercise, and that systolic blood pressure during exercise is kept lower than 200 mm Hg.[14] However, in a clinical trial of older people with renal disease, including 10 with diabetic nephropathy, subjects were treated with a low-protein diet and randomized to 12 weeks of high-intensity resistance training or an inactive control group. The resistance training group had significant improvement in muscle mass, nutritional status, functional capacity, and glomerular filtration rate, which suggests that resistance exercise could be beneficial to patients with diabetic nephropathy.[14]

THE OLDER ATHLETE AND CARDIAC CONDITIONS

Normal aging is associated with diffuse structural and functional changes throughout the cardiovascular system, including increased arterial stiffness, progressive rise in systolic blood pressure, increased pulse pressure, increased impedance to left ventricular ejection, increase in myocardial work and oxygen requirements, increased left atrial size, impaired responsiveness to β_1-adrenergic stimulation, decline in the maximum heart rate, decreased stroke volume and cardiac output, impaired endothelium-mediated vasodilatation, and decreased peak coronary blood flow.[15] These changes contribute to a progressive rise in the incidence and prevalence of cardiovascular disease with increasing age and maintain cardiovascular diseases as the leading cause of death in the United States.[16]

Exercise has proven beneficial for the prevention and treatment of cardiovascular diseases,[5] but older athletes are still at risk of ischemic cardiac events. Sudden cardiac death during exercise is rare, with an incidence rate of 0.54 per 100,000 participants in a study that examined population of 10.9 million runners,[17] but it is still a real concern to many older athletes. The risk of sudden cardiac death approximately doubles during physical activity until about 1 hour after its cessation.[18] There is a consensus that health benefits of regular physical exercise far outweigh the acutely increased risk of sudden cardiac death.[19] In older athletes, atherosclerotic coronary artery disease accounts for more than 80% of sports-related sudden cardiac death and the risk increases with the age of the athlete.[18] To allow the patient to achieve the maximum benefit of activity, while minimizing the risks, one should try to identify patients at risk of coronary artery disease and prescribe individually tailored exercise regimens.

Precompetence screening should help detect individuals at risk for cardiac events, but the efficacy of the various recommended screening methods has not been proven.[18] The screening should include a complete medical history and review of systems, including medications and supplements used by the athlete and toxic habits, such as smoking or alcohol use. The most recent American College of Sports Medicine recommendations for preparticipation health screening eliminate the cardiovascular disease risk factor assessment and risk classification that was previously used. Instead, these new recommendations focus on (1) the individual's current level of physical activity; (2) presence of signs or symptoms of known cardiovascular, metabolic, or renal disease; and (3) the desired exercise intensity, because these variables have been identified as risk modulators of exercise-related cardiovascular events.[20] Individuals are referred to health care providers for medical clearance, which is defined as the approval from a health care professional to engage in exercise, on the basis of the presence of signs or symptoms and/or known cardiovascular, metabolic, or renal disease and physical activity status. The health care provider who gives the medical clearance decides what evaluation, if any, is appropriate before the initiation of a moderate- to vigorous-intensity exercise program.[20]

The American College of Cardiology published in 2005 the 36th Bethesda Conference Report giving specific recommendations for the competitive athletes with cardiovascular abnormalities.[3] For the patient with coronary artery disease they recommend to differentiate between mildly increased and substantially increased risk. Those found with impaired left ventricle systolic function at rest (ie, ejection fraction <50%), evidence of exercise-induced myocardial ischemia, or complex ventricular arrhythmias or hemodynamically significant stenosis of a major coronary artery on angiography should be restricted to low-intensity competitive sports, such as golf, bowling, or billiards.[3] It is also important to educate patients about symptoms of cardiac events, such as chest, arm, jaw, and shoulder discomfort or unusual dyspnea and to instruct them to cease their sport promptly and visit the emergency room as soon as symptoms are detected.

The routine use of a 12-lead electrocardiogram and stress testing in the preparticipation screening of older athletes has been proposed by some authors but remains controversial.[21,22] Exercise testing is considered a poor predictor of acute cardiovascular events, such as heart attacks and sudden death in asymptomatic individuals, because such testing detects flow-limiting coronary lesions, whereas sudden cardiac death and acute myocardial infarction are produced usually by the rapid progression of a previously nonobstructive lesion.[23] Still, further cardiac evaluation should be considered in a patient with a personal history of exertional chest pain or discomfort, unexplained syncope or presyncope, excessive exertional or unexplained dyspnea/fatigue, previous recognition of a heart murmur, and/or an elevated blood pressure.[24] Other red flags to consider further cardiac evaluations include a family history of premature death (sudden and unexpected); a close relative on disability from heart disease before age 50; or the knowledge of family members with hypertrophic or dilated cardiomyopathy, long QT syndrome, ion channelopathies, Marfan syndrome, or clinically important arrhythmias.

Long-term vigorous endurance training is associated with a low prevalence of hypertension[25] but still some older athletes suffer from this chronic condition. Athletes with prehypertension (120–139/80–89 mm Hg) and stage 1 hypertension (140–159/90–99 mm Hg), in the absence of target organ damage, should not be restricted from participation in sports activities. Athletes with stage 2 hypertension (>160/>100 mm Hg) should be restricted from static high-resistance sports (eg, weight training) and should likely be restricted from high-intensity sports until their blood pressure is normalized.[25]

Atrial fibrillation is the most common arrhythmia in clinical practice and the risk of developing this problem in athletes might be significantly higher than in nonathletes. A meta-analysis evaluated the epidemiology of this condition and showed a prevalence of 23% among athletes versus 12.5% in control subjects in a predominantly male population.[26] Atrial ectopic beats, chronic systemic inflammation, autonomic system alterations, anatomic adaptation, myocardial injury, and illicit drugs have been proposed as possible causes for this increased risk.[27] Some athletes experience a reduction of atrial fibrillation attacks by reducing their sporting activity,[28] but others may require cardiology management with drug treatments and even catheter ablation. Direct-current cardioversion is indicated in athletes with atrial fibrillation who require emergency cardioversion caused by hemodynamic instability.[26]

The American College of Cardiology Bethesda Conference recommendations allow athletes with asymptomatic atrial fibrillation, in the absence of structural heart disease, to participate in competitive sports as long as they maintain a ventricular rate that increases and decreases in response to level of activity in a way comparable with that of a normal sinus rhythm while receiving no therapy with atrial ventricular nodal blocking drugs.[3]

THE OLDER ATHLETE AND OSTEOARTHRITIS

Osteoarthritis is the most common joint disorder in the United States affecting nearly 27 million people.[29] This number is likely to increase because of the aging of the population, because age is a one of the strongest risk factors for osteoarthritis.[30] Physical exercise is the most recommended nonpharmacologic intervention for osteoarthritis patients as there is evidence that physical exercise reduces pain and enhances physical function of joints affected by osteoarthritis.[31] An increase of upper leg strength, a decrease of extension impairments, and improvement in proprioception have been proposed as possible causes for the positive association between physical exercise and knee osteoarthritis symptoms.[32]

The possible cause and effect relationship between exercise and osteoarthritis in the elderly is still controversial.[33] Although studies indicate that exercise and physical activity may have a generally positive effect on healthy cartilage metrics, the risk of osteoarthritis development does seem to be moderately increased with sporting participation.[32,34] Joint injury associated with sports participation may be largely responsible for this increased risk. Participation in sports that cause minimal joint impact and torsional loading (walking, swimming, golf, stationary cycling, Tai Chi, water, or low-impact aerobics) may cause osteophyte formation, but should not increase the risk of osteoarthritis in people with normal joints and neuromuscular function. Sports that subject joints to high levels of impact and torsional loading (baseball, lacrosse, basketball, volleyball, soccer, football, rugby, handball, racquetball, tennis, competitive running) increase the risk of injury-induced joint degeneration.[35] The risk is further increased in athletes with abnormal joint anatomy or alignment, previous joint injury or surgery, joint instability, articular surface incongruity or dysplasia, disturbances of joint or muscle innervation, or inadequate muscle strength.[35]

Patients with knee and hip osteoarthritis usually avoid weight-bearing sports activity because of pain. The use of heat therapy in the affected joint before the athletic activity and cold therapy after is commonly recommended for pain control. Also it is advisable to discuss weight loss in overweight and obese patients because the excessive weight is an important modifiable risk factor for osteoarthritis.[36]

THE OLDER ATHLETE AND DEHYDRATION

Dehydration, a form of malnutrition, is a significant concern in the older athlete. Decreased thirst response and a reduced kidney function increase the risk of dehydration in this group, especially when exercising in extreme temperatures. Also, the thermoregulation and sweating mechanism is affected with age.[37] Social reasons, such as fear of incontinence or the lack of availability of a toilet, may cause some older people to restrict their fluid intake and predispose them further to dehydration.

Athletes often dehydrate involuntarily during exercise when fluid losses exceed replacement. It is a commonly accepted practice to weigh before and after exercise to monitor hydration, although urine concentration test provides a more accurate measurement. A body water deficit of greater than 2% of body weight marks the level of dehydration that negatively affects not only sports performance, but also short-term memory, working memory, and psychomotor and visual motor skills. Extreme cases of dehydration can lead to the development of heat exhaustion, exertional heat stroke, and/or acute renal failure consequent to exertional rhabdomyolysis.[38,39]

There are various general prescriptive guidelines for fluid and electrolyte replacement for athletes. However, it is difficult to recommend a specific fluid and electrolyte replacement schedule that fits every athlete because of considerable variability in the type of exercise, metabolic requirements, duration, clothing, equipment, weather conditions; and personal factors, such as genetic predisposition, heat acclimatization, and training status. To start the sport activity with an adequate hydration, it is recommended to start prehydration at least several hours before the exercise task to enable fluid absorption and allow urine output to return toward normal levels. During the competition athletes should continue the intake of fluids to avoid excessive dehydration. Opportunities to drink and availability of fluids are influenced by the culture and rules of the sport.[38]

Older athletes often present slower excretion of water and electrolytes, therefore increasing the risk of hyponatremia with excess water and the risk of hypertension as a result of excess sodium ingestion. This should be discussed with the competitor because, although dehydration is more common, overdrinking with a consequent symptomatic hyponatremia is considered more dangerous. Intravenous fluid replacement may be required in athletes who develop nausea, vomiting, or diarrhea, or in those who for some reason cannot ingest fluids, but serum sodium level should be checked before attempting aggressive fluid replacement.[39]

USE OF COMMON MEDICATIONS IN THE OLDER ATHLETE

The use of medications and dietary supplements is common among the older population and among athletes.[40] When treating older athletes, it is important to consider and discuss in detail with the patient the use of medications and the potential effects of drugs in sports performance and overall health condition.

For example, nonsteroidal anti-inflammatory drugs are one of the most commonly used drug classes, currently available over the counter. Their use is popular among athletes to treat pain and its use is reported to increase with age.[41] This group of medications has been found to increase the risk of gastrointestinal bleeding or peptic ulcer disease, especially in patients older than 75 years of age and those taking oral or parenteral corticosteroids, anticoagulants, or antiplatelet agents. Upper gastrointestinal ulcers, gross bleeding, or perforation caused by nonsteroidal anti-inflammatory drugs occur in approximately 1% of patients treated for 3 to 6 months and approximately 2% to 4% of patients treated for 1 year.[42] The use of nonsteroidal anti-inflammatory drugs is also associated with a potential increased risk of cardiovascular complications[43] and renal complications, including sodium and water retention with edema, worsening of heart failure, hypertension, hyponatremia, hyperkalemia, acute kidney injury, chronic kidney disease, renal papillary necrosis, and acute interstitial nephritis.[44] Risks increase with the potential dehydration that can occur during a sports competition. Skeletal muscle relaxants should be avoided in older athletes because they are often poorly tolerated due to anticholinergic adverse effects, sedation, and increased risk of fractures.[42]

Many older athletes also use medications for cardiovascular conditions. Diuretics, commonly prescribed for hypertension, increase the risks of dehydration and electrolyte imbalance. β-Adrenergic blocking agents can impair performance during participation in intense competitive sports.[45] Nitrates may cause orthostatic hypotension; calcium channel blockers and α-adrenergic agents can also cause bradycardia.[42] Athletes who require anticoagulation should not participate in sports in which there is danger of trauma or bodily collision.[3] Statins are another commonly prescribed medication among the older population. This group of medications is known to cause mild muscle complaints including myalgia, cramps, and weakness with or without creatine kinase elevations.[46] These symptoms are usually reversible and more likely to occur in older adults.[47] Treatment with coenzyme Q10 (200 mg daily) seems to improve muscle performance in older athletes taking statins.[48]

Finally, the use of dietary supplements should be discussed with older athletes. It is estimated that at least 60% of all athletes consume these products,[49] but it is possible that the number is higher for older populations. Many of the commonly used products have not been thoroughly studied and may have unknown adverse effects. Some dietary supplements may not be safe because of poor quality control by manufacturers, inadequate storage conditions, or deliberate addition of unknown components to increase the efficacy of the product.[49] This last factor is particularly important for master athletes participating in official competitions because some of these components may be banned by the World Anti-Doping Agency and may cause disqualification of the athlete.

REFERENCES

1. Available at: http://nsga.com/30history. Accessed April 12, 2017.
2. Brun SP. Clinical considerations for the ageing athlete. Aust Fam Physician 2016; 45(7):478–83.
3. Maron BJ, Zipes D. 36th Bethesda Conference: eligibility recommendations for competitive athletes with cardiovascular abnormalities. J Am Coll Cardiol 2005; 45(8):1314–75.
4. Available at: http://www.itftennis.com/seniors/world-individual-championships/overview/overview.aspx. Accessed April 1, 2017.
5. Chodzko-Zajko WJ, Proctor DN, Fiatarone Singh M, et al. American College of Sports Medicine position stand. Exercise and physical activity for older adults. Med Sci Sports Exerc 2009;41(7):1510–30.

6. Kettunen JA, Kujala UM, Kaprio J, et al. Health of master track and field athletes: a 16-year follow-up study. Clin J Sport Med 2006;16(2):142–8.

7. Available at: https://www.cdc.gov/diabetes/pdfs/data/2014-report-estimates-of-diabetes-and-its-burden-in-the-united-states.pdf. Accessed March 16, 2017.

8. Ryan AS. Exercise in aging: its important role in mortality, obesity and insulin resistance. Aging Health 2010;6(5):551–63.

9. Seals DR, Hagberg JM, Hurley BE, et al. Glucose tolerance in young and older athletes and sedentary men. J Appl Physiol 1984;56:1521–5.

10. Pratley RE, Hagberg JM, Rogus EM, et al. Enhanced insulin sensitivity and lower waist-to-hip ratio in master athletes. Am J Physiol 1995;268:E484–90.

11. Tuomilehto J, Lindström J, Eriksson JG, Finnish Diabetes Prevention Study Group. Prevention of type 2 diabetes mellitus by changes in lifestyle among subjects with impaired glucose tolerance. N Engl J Med 2001;344(18):1343–50.

12. Kirk SE. The diabetic athlete. In: Miller M, Thompson SR, editors. DeLee & Drez's orthopaedic sports medicine. 4th edition. Philadelphia (PA): Elsevier Saunders; 2014. p. 242–50.

13. Sigal RJ, Kenny GP, Wasserman DH, et al. Physical activity and type 2 diabetes. Diabetes Care 2004;27(10):2518–39.

14. Castaneda C, Gordon PL, Uhlin KL. Resistance training to counteract the catabolism of a low-protein diet in patients with chronic renal insufficiency: a randomized, controlled trial. Ann Intern Med 2001;135(11):965–76.

15. Stolker JM, Rich MW. Aging and heart disease. In: Crawford MH, DiMarco JP, Paulus WJ, editors. Cardiology. 3rd edition. Philadelphia: Mosby Elsevier Ltd; 2010. p. 1775–90.

16. Available at: https://www.cdc.gov/nchs/fastats/leading-causes-of-death.htm. Accessed March 19, 2017.

17. Kim JH, Malhotra R, Chiampas G, et al. Cardiac arrest during long-distance running races. N Engl J Med 2012;366(2):130–40.

18. Schmied C, Borjesson M. Sudden cardiac death in athletes. J Intern Med 2014; 275:93–103.

19. Thompson PD, Franklin BA, Balady GJ, et al. Exercise and acute cardiovascular events. Placing the risks into perspective. A scientific statement from the American heart Association Council on nutrition, physical activity, and metabolism and the Council on Clinical Cardiology. Circulation 2007;115:2358–68.

20. Riebe D, Franklin B, Thompson P, et al. Updating ACSMs recommendations for exercise preparticipation health screening. Med Sci Sports Exerc 2015;47(11): 2473–9.

21. Corrado D, Basso C, Thiene G. Sudden cardiac death in athletes: what is the role of screening? Curr Opin Cardiol 2012;27(1):41–8.

22. Schmied CM. Improvement of cardiac screening in amateur athletes. J Electrocardiol 2015;48(3):351–5.

23. Thompson PD, Arena R, Riebe D, et al. ACSM's New Preparticipation Health Screening Recommendations from ACSM's Guidelines for Exercise Testing and Prescription, Ninth Edition. Curr Sports Med Rep 2013;12(4):215–7.

24. American Academy of Family Physicians, American Academy of Orthopaedic Surgeons, American College of Sports Medicine; American Medical Society for Sports Medicine, American Orthopaedic Society for Sports Medicine, American Osteopathic Academy of Sports Medicine, Kibler WB, Putukian M. Selected issues for the master athlete and the team physician: a consensus statement. Med Sci Sports Exerc 2010;42(4):820–33.

25. Hernelahti M, Kujala UM, Kaprio J, et al. Hypertension in master endurance athletes. J Hypertens 1998;16(11):1573–7.
26. Abdulla J, Nielsen JR. Is the risk of atrial fibrillation higher in athletes than in the general population? A systematic review and meta-analysis. Europace 2009;11:1156–9.
27. Goudis CA, Ntalas JV, Ketikoglou DG. Atrial fibrillation in athletes. Cardiol Rev 2015;23:247–51.
28. Hoogsteena J, Schepb G, van Hemelc NM, et al. Paroxysmal atrial fibrillation in male endurance athletes. A 9-year follow up. Europace 2004;6(3):222–8.
29. Lawrence RC, Felson DT, Helmick CG, et al. Estimates of the prevalence of arthritis and other rheumatic conditions in the United States: Part II. Arthritis Rheum 2008;58(1):26–35.
30. Zhang Y, Jordan JM. Epidemiology of osteoarthritis. Clin Geriatr Med 2010;26:355–69.
31. Tanaka R, Ozawa J, Kito N, et al. Efficacy of strengthening or aerobic exercise on pain relief in people with knee osteoarthritis: a systematic review and meta-analysis of randomized controlled trials. Clin Rehabil 2013;27(12):1059–71.
32. Runhaar J, Luijsterburg P, Dekker J, et al. Identifying potential working mechanisms behind the positive effects of exercise therapy on pain and function in osteoarthritis; a systematic review. Osteoarthritis Cartilage 2015;23(7):1071–82.
33. Tran G, Smith TO, Grice A, et al. Does sports participation (including level of performance and previous injury) increase risk of osteoarthritis? A systematic review and meta-analysis. Br J Sports Med 2016;50(23):1459–66.
34. Bennell K, Hinman RS, Wrigley TV, et al. Exercise and osteoarthritis: cause and effects. Compr Physiol 2011;1(4):1943–2008.
35. Buckwalter JA, Martin JA. Sports and osteoarthritis. Curr Opin Rheumatol 2004;16(5):634–9.
36. Yusuf E, Nelissen RG, Ioan-Facsinay A, et al. Association between weight or body mass index and hand osteoarthritis: a systematic review. Ann Rheum Dis 2010;69(4):761–5.
37. Blatteis CM. Age-dependent changes in temperature regulation: a mini review. Gerontology 2012;58(4):289–95.
38. American College of Sports Medicine, Sawka MN, Burke LM, et al. American College of Sports Medicine position stand. Exercise and fluid replacement. Med Sci Sports Exerc 2007;39(2):377–90.
39. Casa DJ, Clarkson PM, Roberts WO. American College of Sports Medicine Roundtable on hydration and physical activity: consensus statements. Curr Sports Med Rep 2005;4:115–27.
40. Suzic Lazic J, Dikic N, Radivojevic N, et al. Dietary supplements and medications in elite sport: polypharmacy or real need? Scand J Med Sci Sports 2011;21(2):260–7.
41. Wehling M. Non-steroidal anti-inflammatory drug use in chronic pain conditions with special emphasis on the elderly and patients with relevant comorbidities: management and mitigation of risks and adverse effects. Eur J Clin Pharmacol 2014;70:1159–72.
42. American Geriatrics Society 2015 Beers Criteria Update Expert Panel. American Geriatrics Society 2015 updated Beers criteria for potentially inappropriate medication use in older adults. J Am Geriatr Soc 2015;63(11):2227–46.
43. Fanelli A, Romualdi P, Vigano' R, et al. Non-selective non-steroidal anti-inflammatory drugs (NSAIDs) and cardiovascular risk. Acta Biomed 2013;84(1):5–11.

44.Ković SV, Vujović KS, Srebro D, et al. Prevention of renal complications induced by non- steroidal anti-inflammatory drugs. Curr Med Chem 2016;23(19):1953–64.
45. Maron BJ, Araújo CG, Thompson PD, et al. Recommendations for preparticipation screening and the assessment of cardiovascular disease in masters athletes. An advisory for healthcare professionals from the Working Groups of the World Heart Federation, the International Federation of Sports Medicine, and the American Heart Association Committee on Exercise, Cardiac Rehabilitation, and Prevention. Circulation 2001;103:327–34.
46. Taylor BA, Thompson PD. Muscle-related side-effects of statins: from mechanisms to evidence-based solutions. Curr Opin Lipidol 2015;26(3):221–7.
47. Cham S, Evans MA, Denenberg JO, et al. Statin-associated muscle related adverse effects: a case series of 354 patients. Pharmacotherapy 2010;30(6): 541–53.
48. Deichmann RE, Lavie CJ, Dornelles AC. Impact of coenzyme Q-10 on parameters of cardiorespiratory fitness and muscle performance in older athletes taking statins. Phys Sportsmed 2012;40(4):88–95.
49. Deldicque L, Francaux M. Potential harmful effects of dietary supplements in sports medicine. Curr Opin Clin Nutr Metab Care 2016;19(6):439–45.

Musculoskeletal Injuries and Regenerative Medicine in the Elderly Patient

John C. Cianca, MD[a],*, Prathap Jayaram, MD[b]

KEYWORDS

- Regenerative medicine • Platelet-rich plasma • Stem cell therapy • Prolotherapy
- Osteoarthritis

KEY POINTS

- Regenerative medicine is an emerging field that has value in musculoskeletal injuries and conditions in the elderly.
- Viscosupplementation and prolotherapy are established therapies that continue to show efficacy in the elderly population.
- Platelet-rich plasma injections and mesenchymal stem cell therapy are emerging therapeutic strategies that have shown a good safety profile.

INTRODUCTION

Regenerative medicine has gained increasing popularity in its clinical applications, particularly in the field of musculoskeletal medicine. Regenerative medicine, a broad term, can be thought of as a particular medical strategy that strives to rebuild and restore diseased tissue to normal physiologic tissue baseline. Simply put, regenerative strategies augment the body's innate physiology to heal pathologic processes.[1] This article focuses on specific regenerative strategies and the uses of them for common pathologies in the aging adult, including platelet-rich plasma (PRP), mesenchymal stem cells (MSCs), viscosupplementation, and prolotherapy.

COMMON CONDITIONS AFFECTING THE ELDERLY
Tendinopathy

Tendinopathy is common degenerative condition seen in all adults, but in particular in tendons of the elderly. Tendinopathy is thought to result primarily from a blunted

The authors have nothing to disclose.
[a] Department of Physical Medicine and Rehabiltation, Baylor College of Medicine, University of Texas Health Science Center, 1 Baylor Plaza, Houston, TX 77030, USA; [b] Department of Physical Medicine and Rehabiltation and Orthopedic Surgery, Regenerative Sports Medicine, Baylor College of Medicine, 1 Baylor Plaza, Houston, TX 77030, USA
* Corresponding author. Human Performance Center, 5959 West Loop South, Suite 260, Bellaire, TX 77401.
E-mail address: john.cianca@hpchouston.com

inflammatory response to tendonitis, leading to a degenerative cycle of abnormal healing.[2] Chronic repetitive tendon overload is the most commonly proposed theory, with high loads causing microscopic alterations at the cellular level that weaken the mechanical properties. Aging can result in progressive loss of mobility with subsequent deterioration in quality of life. A major component of this loss of mobility is progressive muscle weakness, as elderly muscles become smaller, more susceptible to damage, and regenerate and recover more slowly than in their youth.[3] Only recently has it been recognized that, in addition to skeletal muscle changes, alterations in tendon properties contribute to muscle weakness and loss of mobility in old age.[3]

Rotator cuff tendinopathy

Rotator cuff tendinopathy is the most common cause of shoulder pain in all age groups, accounting for 30% of shoulder related pain.[4] It arises from the repetitive strain incurred by overuse and poor postural control because the rotator cuff acts in its role as the primary dynamic stabilizer of the glenohumeral joint. Clinical features of rotator cuff tendinopathy include pain, crepitus, and increased pain with overhead activities of daily living. In a study done by Milgrom and colleagues,[5] the prevalence of RTC tears markedly increased after 50 years of age, with more than 50% of dominant shoulders in the seventh decade and 80% of subjects greater than 80 years of age. Riley and colleagues[6] demonstrated that the supraspinatus tendon undergoes a decrease in glycosaminoglycan, chondroitin sulfate and dermatan sulfate with age. In another study by Rudzki and colleagues,[7] regional variations in supraspinatus tendon vascularity were shown in an age-dependent manner. These results support that, even without clinical symptoms, the aging shoulder is likely to transition to attritional tendinopathy, perhaps making the shoulder more susceptible to injury.

Gluteal tendinopathy

Gluteal tendinopathy commonly presents as pain and tenderness laterally over the greater trochanter (lateral hip pain). It is a cause of moderate to severe pain and disability,[8–11] with 1 study demonstrating quality of life and levels of disability similar to those in end-stage hip osteoarthritis (OA).[12] Gluteal tendinopathy is most prevalent in women aged greater than 40 years[13,14] with reports of up to 23.5% of women and 8.5% of men between the ages of 50 and 79 years being afflicted with condition.[14] It is the most prevalent of all lower limb tendinopathies.[15] The mechanism leading to its development is multifactorial. Load shear strain, as mentioned, is a particular contributing factor. The influence of joint position affects compressive tendon loading from excessive hip adduction.[16] Patients with gluteal tendinopathy may experience pain after prolonged sitting, with subsequent difficulty in rising to standing, particularly if they have been sitting with more than 90° of hip flexion in a low lounge or car seat. Surrounding muscle architecture also plays a role in development of tendon pathology: the tensor fascia lata has been shown to hypertrophy[17] and gluteus medius and gluteus minimus atrophy[18] in those with gluteal tendon pathology. Bone morphology influences the compressive forces at the hip by vectors from the iliotibial band. The typical femoral neck angle of 128°, the iliotibial band exerted a compressive force of 656 N at the greater trochanter, but at 115° (coxa vara), the compressive force was 997 N.[19] These findings suggest that patients with more severe gluteal tendon pathology have lower femoral neck–shaft angles than pain-free controls or those with hip OA.

Knee extensor mechanism tendinopathy

Patellar tendinopathy, also referred to as jumpers knee, results from chronic tendon overuse and overload of the knee extensor mechanism. The most common location of pain is the superior patellar pole for the quadriceps tendon and the inferior patellar pole in the patellar tendon. The exact etiology is not well-established; however, it is thought to be due in part to peripheral peritendinous pain receptors or the neovascularization that occurs after injury.[20,21] Risk factors are thought to include poor hamstring and quadriceps flexibility, poor knee joint coordination, reduced ankle dorsiflexion, and increased pronation velocity of the foot.[22] There is some controversy regarding how aging affects patellar tendon collagen cross-linking. Couppe and colleagues[23] showed that human patellar tendon collagen concentration was reduced, whereas cross-linking of concentration was elevated in elderly men versus younger men, which may be a mechanism to maintain the mechanical properties of tendon with aging. Another study looking at aging effects on patellar tendon showed that patellar tendon mechanical properties at maximal force are altered with aging, and these differences are more related to force output rather than to an age effect.[24]

Achilles tendinopathy Achilles tendinopathy is a common clinical condition that affects the elderly and is characterized by pain and swelling in the middle and distal portions of the Achilles tendon. The development of tendinopathy once again is thought to be due to overuse and repetitive loading. Intrinsic risk factors in the elderly are thought to be decreased ankle dorsiflexion range of motion, abnormal subtalar range of motion, decreased plantar flexion strength, excessive foot pronation, and poor tendon vascularity.[25] Recent work in ultrasound using elastography has shown increased stiffness in elderly subjects, which may be a contributing factor for the high prevalence of Achilles tendinopathy observed in elderly patients.[26]

Degenerative Joint Disease

OA is a common clinical condition with a prevalence of 40 million people in the United States. More than 80% of individuals over the age of 55 have radiographic evidence of OA. Among those, 30% of the individuals present with significant pain or disabilities.[27] This equates to 5.6 million individuals in the United States and corresponds with an annual expenditure of $3 billion for posttraumatic arthritis.[28] However, current treatment of OA is limited to lifestyle modification, analgesics, and invasive procedures such as joint replacement surgery in severe cases. The mechanism and important biological contributors in OA remain largely unknown. Therefore, new clinical strategies that may improve the evaluation and augment repair and regeneration of damaged articular cartilage that prevent or delay the onset of disabling pain and OA have become a increasingly prevalent clinical strategy.

Degenerative Disc Disease

Increases in life expectancy will lead to a higher number of elderly people.[29] According to the United Nations Population Fund, people aged 60 years and older made up more than 11% of the global population in 2012, a proportion that will increase to about 22% by 2050.[30] Consequently, physicians will face an ever-increasing number of elderly patients suffering from degenerative processes such as degenerative disc disease in the future. Low back pain is a very common cause of pain in the elderly that affects up to 80% of adults at some time during their life. In people over 55 years of age, 95% of lumbar disc herniations occur at the L4 to L5 and L5 to S1 levels.[31–34] Early nonoperative intervention is always attempted first; however, there are cases where surgical intervention is necessary. Long-term outcomes after surgery remain a controversial topic, which has created a role for regenerative strategies.

Spinal Stenosis

Lumbar spinal stenosis refers to narrowing of the lumbar spinal canal either centrally, laterally, or at the neural foramina. The narrowing is associated with neural compression, and clinically most often manifests fatigue with walking or standing, weakness, or radicular pain in 1 or both legs. Lumbar spinal stenosis has an annual incidence of near 5 per 100,000.[35] The prevalence increases with age, and is suggested to be between 1.7% and 8.0% in the general elderly population.[35] It is the most common diagnosis leading to spinal surgery in patients over the age of 65. Approximately 1 in 1000 people over the age of 65 have had a laminectomy for lumbar spinal stenosis, with an estimated cost of $1 billion.[36] There are no regenerative strategies to date that target the central stenosis etiology, but surrounding structural changes of facet arthrosis have been targeted.

REGENERATIVE TREATMENT STRATEGIES FOR MUSCULOSKELETAL CONDITIONS
Viscosupplementation: Historical Perspective and Use

Hyaluronate is a naturally occurring component of the cartilage and the synovial fluid. It is a polysaccharide composed of continuously repeating molecular sequences of β-D-glucuronic acid and β-d-N-acetylglucosamine, with a molecular mass in normal synovial fluid ranging from 6500 to 10,900 kDa.[37] Within the normal adult knee, there is approximately 2 mL of synovial fluid, with a hyaluronate concentration of 2.5 to 4.0 mg/mL.[38] Hyaluronate is responsible for lubricating and potentially reducing shear forces within the knee joint, depending on the forces exerted on it.[39] In OA, synovial hyaluronate is depolymerized and cleared at higher rates than normal.[40] In a normal joint, the average intrasynovial half-life of hyaluronate is approximately 20 hours.[38] In an inflamed joint, this half-life is decreased to 11 to 12 hours. These changes reduce the viscoelasticity of the synovial fluid.

Viscosupplementation is an exogenous hyaluronate that was developed as a treatment for the symptoms of knee OA. Viscosupplementation can be thought of as a first-generation biologic strategy; it can be either synthesized by means of bacterial fermentation or extracted from animal tissues (eg, rooster comb). The therapeutic goal of administration of intraarticular hyaluronate is to provide and maintain intraarticular lubrication, and increase the viscoelastic properties of synovial fluid[41]; Another proposed mechanism is that hyaluronate exerts antiinflammatory, analgesic, and possibly chondroprotective effects on the articular cartilage and joint synovium.[38] The clinical benefits of treatment with intraarticular hyaluronate, which persist well beyond the intraarticular residence time of the product, have been suggested to be caused by the reestablishment of joint homeostasis as a result of an increase in the endogenous production of hyaluronate that persists long after the exogenous injected material has left the joint.[40]

There is no clear supporting evidence of clinical criteria to select patients who will likely benefit from hyaluronate injections. However, trial data suggest that patients with late-stage disease (such as those with marked joint space narrowing) who are older than 65 years of age are less likely than younger patients or patients with earlier disease to have any benefit, that is, the lower the grading in the Kellgren Lawrence scale, the greater the effect of viscosupplementation.[42]

Tenotomy

A mechanical treatment technique that is used primarily for tendons, tenotomy is analogous to trigger point work in muscles. It is alternatively referred to as tendon fenestration or dry needling. The goal is to target pathologic changes within a tendon with the intention of initiating a healing response. A hypodermic needle is introduced into the tendon guided by ultrasound imaging. The needle is repeatedly advanced and withdrawn within the pathologic portion of the tendon. Ultrasonographic guidance allows the needle to be placed precisely within the area of pathology. This is done by viewing the needle in plane first as it enters the tissue. Once localized to the area of pathology, the ultrasonographic transducer is turned 90° out of plane with the needle, providing a cross-sectional view of the pathologic area. The needling action is continued in a back and forth motion with redirection across the width of the area of pathology, as seen with the transducer. The needle is out of plane with the transducer and only the tip is seen as it advances in and out of the tissue (**Figs. 1** and **2**). This process introduces injury to the tendon tissue, invoking bleeding and an acute inflammatory response in the region. If the area of pathology is in an enthesis, then the bony insertion is needled as well. The needle action causes bleeding from both tissues and this mechanism of injury induces an acute inflammatory reaction mediated by a variety of growth factors and in so doing the tendon may be able to remodel and heal.[43] Tenotomy is frequently used with other regenerative techniques, such as prolotherapy and PRP. These entities further support a healing process by providing substrates locally to the tendon, which often has a limited blood supply. Compared with surgical treatment, it is less expensive and has a lower rate of associated adverse events. Tenotomy proved effective for reducing pain in lateral epicondylosis and several other tendinopathies.[44]

A retrospective study 82% of patients treated with tendon fenestration for tendinopathy of the gluteus medius, minimus, proximal hamstring, or the tensor fascia lata showed marked improvement.[45] The tendon fenestration technique has been demonstrated to be effective in a prospective study on a variety of tendinopathic conditions measuring pain using a visual analog scale.[46]

Tenotomy has been shown to be effective used alone for treatment when compared with its use with steroid.[47] In another study, PRP with tenotomy had a greater effect initially but was no more effective than tenotomy alone after 6 months.[48]

Other needle techniques that have been reported to have a reparative effect on tendinopathy include tendon scraping[49] to disrupt neovascular tissue and the associated nerve ingrowth into chronically affected tendons. Disrupting these nerves is thought to have a pain-relieving effect. Using shock waves and rapidly oscillating percutaneous needling has also been shown to have similar effects as needle fenestration.[50]

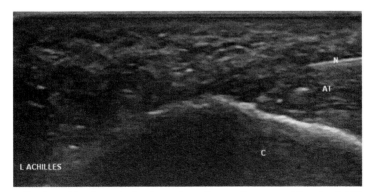

Fig. 1. Needle viewed in plane. An in-plane view of a needle approaching the Achilles tendon insertion during a tenotomy. AT, Achilles tendon; C, calcaneus; N, Needle. *Courtesy of* John C Cianca, MD, Baylor College of Medicine, University of Texas Health Science Center, Houston, TX.

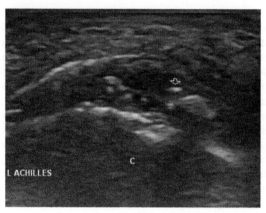

Fig. 2. Needle viewed out of plane. An out-of-plane view of a needle in the Achilles tendon during a tenotomy. C, calcaneus; arrow head, needle tip. *Courtesy of* John C Cianca, MD, Baylor College of Medicine, University of Texas Health Science Center, Houston, TX.

Prolotherapy

Prolotherapy as it is now known originally was called sclerotherapy. Sclerotherapy had its origins in 16th century France. Chemical irritants were injected into incompetent or lax ligaments resulting in fibrous tissue formation (scar) and promoting structural stability in the tissue.[51] Hackett[52] began using less noxious injectants in the mid-20th century resulting in proliferation of the affected tissue. He began referring to this technique as prolotherapy so as to differentiate it from the sclerotherapy technique. Prolotherapy evolved during the later decades of the 20th century and during the early years of the 21st century.[52] Hackett's original research demonstrated an increase in the size of tendon and tendon enthesis in an animal model 2 weeks after treatment.[53] As the treatment technique has evolved, it has been used more liberally in a variety of tissues and conditions. Early formulations included synasol and sodium murrhuate and a formula of phenol, glycerin, and glucose.[54] Dextrose is the agent of choice in current clinical practice. Local anesthetic as well as sterile water or normal saline are added to 50% dextrose creating formulas with as high as 25% dextrose and as low as 5% dextrose.

It is commonly believed that these proliferants cause an osmotic gradient with the target tissue leading to cell desiccation and an inflammatory response. Growth factors are released within the tissues as a result, leading to a healing response.[55,56] Furthermore, it is postulated that dextrose serves as a signaling agent in tendon repair.[55] As such, it may be considered the first injectable regenerative medicine agent.

As a prerequisite, the patient should be withdrawn from nonsteroidal antiinflammatory drugs for 2 to 3 days before treatment to allow the inflammatory response to be initiated. The injection technique uses small gauge needles, generally 25 to 30 gauge, advancing into and around the tissue. Once in the tissue, a tenotomy-like action is often used followed by injection of the dextrose solution in small aliquots (less than 1 mL per site). Additionally, where applicable, bone stimulation is done. This has been postulated to result in additional release of chemical mediators of injury. The upregulation of a variety of growth factors specific to ligaments and tendons as well as cartilage have been identified.[57] When accurately delivered, the treatment is safe and only minimally painful. After the procedure, patients may have soreness or mild to moderate pain owing to the induction of an inflammatory response. Resting the affected tissue from impact and repetitive use or loading is recommended. Gentle passive or active assisted motions are encouraged. Nonnarcotic pain relievers such as acetaminophen are usually sufficient if needed. Nonsteroidal antiinflammatory drugs should be avoided for 7 to 10 days.

Back pain is prevalent in middle-aged and senior adults. OA of the spine, degenerative disc disease, and spinal stenosis are all prevalent diagnoses. Sacroiliac joint, coccydynia, and ligamentous causes of back pain are also common. Prolotherapy has been used to treat low back pain for many decades.[52,53,58–60] More recent studies have demonstrated greater duration in pain relief than steroid in the sacroiliac joint.[55] Prolotherapy resulted in extended pain relief in patients with discogenic pain with or without radicular pain in another study.[61]

OA is a significant cause of functional decline and disability. It is also a considerable driver of health care costs in the aging adult. The use of prolotherapy in recent years to treat osteoarthritic joints has had encouraging results. Studies using animal models have demonstrated a chondroprotective effect of intraarticular dextrose injections.[62] Randomized, controlled trials have demonstrated pain reduction and functional improvement in humans.[63–65] Most recently, pain reduction and functional improvement as well as chondrogenesis was demonstrated in a case series.[66] Additionally, studies of have demonstrated clinical improvement in OA of the thumb[63]

Treatment protocols for OA rely on intraarticular injections of dextrose solutions ranging from 12.5% to 25%. Cessation of nonsteroidal antiinflammatory medications before treatment and after treatment is recommended as with other prolotherapy regimens. Rest from weight bearing exercise for several days is encouraged. Treatments are usually administered at monthly intervals for 2 to 4 months.

In addition, adjunctive superficial injections of dextrose solutions may be done along the affected joint surface. Now known as perineural injection therapy, this technique targets superficial nerves in the region of pathology. It is purported that these superficial nerves are responsible for neurogenic inflammation that can cause a chronic upregulation of pain via the activation of transient receptor potential vanilloid 1 channels, leading to chronic pain and soft tissue dysfunction. Injection of 5% dextrose around these nerves can stabilize nerve function reducing neurogenic inflammation.[67]

People in general and older adults in particular have been encouraged to be more active to promote health. However, with an increasing level of activity, there is likely to be a greater incidence of overuse injuries and pathologies. The occurrence of tendon pathology has become clinically relevant. Several studies have been done demonstrating pain relief and functional improvement in patients with common extensor tendon, and patellar and Achilles tendinopathies as well as plantar fasciopathy.[68–72] Prolotherapy compared favorably with PRP in the treatment of chronic plantar fasciitis.[73] A systematic review of several case series and controlled trials found prolotherapy, PRP, polidocanol, and autologous whole blood to be effective in the treatment of lateral epicondylosis.[68] In addition, 1 study demonstrated structural improvement in the patellar tendinopathy.[69]

The safety profile of prolotherapy has been established and, owing to its inexpensive treatment technique, provides an alternative treatment option. It is being used with greater frequency in clinical medicine. Nonetheless, more robust research needs to be done. Although evidence is growing and becoming more substantive, much of the research has been case reports and uncontrolled trials.[74] It has usefulness in a variety of conditions that are common and likely to become more prevalent as people live longer and become more active.

Platelet-Rich Plasma

PRP is a derivative of autologous blood containing a higher than physiologic concentration of platelets.[75] To date, there is no standard protocol for PRP formulations. The efficacy of PRP is, therefore, likely impacted by the composition of the PRP itself. This can lead to high degrees of variability in comparing the efficacy of PRP across clinical studies. Several classification systems for PRP have been proposed, although none have been widely accepted.[76–78] In an attempt to better understand clinical efficacy, this classification has been suggested to categorize the type of PRP injected.[79]

Preparations

PRP preparation requires 15 to 100 mL of whole blood obtained via peripheral venipuncture, depending on the commercial method being used. PRP is prepared by centrifugation of anticoagulated whole blood. It is initially separated into 3 layers based on specific gravity: (1) plasma (top layer), (2) platelets and leukocytes (middle layer, termed the "buffy coat"), and (3) red blood cells (bottom layer). The bottom layer is typically discarded; the buffy coat and top layer are then often subjected to a second centrifugation to separate PRP from platelet-poor plasma. PRP may then be activated with calcium chloride or thrombin to cause the release of growth factors from alpha granules to occur more rapidly, although this additional step is not performed universally. Different harvesting and centrifugation methods yield different volumes and concentrations of platelets.[80] There is also great variability in the timing of PRP acquisition. It has been shown that PRP samples produced from the same patient, using the same centrifugation protocol and equipment, may lead to PRP of varying composition.[81]

Applications

There has been an increase in the usefulness of PRP for degenerative musculoskeletal conditions in the last decade. Given the lack of reported studies characterizing PRP, it becomes difficult to support a specific level of evidence and clinical recommendation. However, there is level 1 evidence to support its use in lateral epicondylosis and tendinopathy, as well as OA of the knee.[82] Although lateral elbow tendinopathy does not affect the elderly population as frequently as younger populations, its degenerative mechanism of tension loading and failure to remodel is akin to other prevalent tendinopathies in the elderly. Corticosteroids, which have been widely used in the past, have been shown to have a deleterious effect on tendon and joint tissue.[83] In contrast, the use of such agents as PRP, which may stimulate tissue healing and have no deleterious effects, seem to be a more reasonable choice. PRP applications to elderly rotator cuff dysfunction has not been supported by high level evidence. However, in recent years there has been an increase in studies involving operative rotator cuff repairs[83–86] and some evidence to support its use in direct treatment of RTC injuries.[87]

In general, evidence for the effectiveness of PRP remains weak. In a prospective, randomized, double-blind study, Weber and colleagues[84] compared recovery from arthroscopic rotator cuff repair with and without application of a platelet-rich fibrin matrix and found no differences in range of motion, pain, and rate of retear at multiple time points up to 12 weeks postoperatively. In another prospective cohort study, Jo and colleagues[85] found that treatment with PRP did not enhance arthroscopic rotator cuff repair in terms of discomfort, strength, movement, function, or satisfaction after 16 months. Similarly, Bergeson and colleagues[86] were unable to show the benefits of a platelet-rich fibrin matrix for arthroscopic rotator cuff repair in comparison with controls. Kesikburun and colleagues[87] compared PRP with saline for the treatment of chronic rotator cuff tendinopathy and found significant improvement in both groups, with sizable improvements in both pain and function. Rha and colleagues[88] compared ultrasound-guided PRP injection with dry needling. Dry needling or 2 PRP injections were performed 4 weeks apart and significant improvement was found in the Shoulder Pain and Disability Index scores, passive internal rotation, and flexion of patients treated with PRP as early as 6 weeks, which continued until 6 months after injection. These studies were not restricted to an elderly population and more conclusive studies need to be done before providing a recommendation.

Studies of gluteal tendinopathy, although highly prevalent in the elderly, has yielded little evidence to support the use of PRP. A recent study by Lee and colleagues[89] studied 21 patients prospectively who all received 1 guided PRP injections for recalcitrant tendinosis and/or partial gluteus medius tears with significant improvement in subjective outcomes. Given how prevalent this pathology is, more robust studies need to be done before this can be recommended strongly.

Patellar tendinopathy has been studied more robustly compared with gluteal tendinopathy, however, not exclusively in the elderly. Kon and colleagues[90] evaluated the effects of a series of 3 PRP injections, each given 15 days apart, with significantly improved overall function, pain, perception of physical and emotional health, vitality, and a sense of limitation at 6 months. James and colleagues[91] looked at the usefulness of 2 injections of autologous blood at 4-week intervals, in combination with dry needling, demonstrating significant improvement in the Victorian Institute of Sports Assessment score at follow-up, which averaged approximately 15 months. In a recent systematic review by Everhart and colleagues,[92] examining 15 studies their conclusion for initial patellar tendinopathy treatment should consist of eccentric squat-based therapy, shockwave, or PRP as monotherapy or an adjunct to accelerate recovery. Reproducible and comparative clinical results are lacking, owing to at least in part to the variety of PRP preparations and treatment methods.

There is an established safety profile for PRP applications in Achilles tendinopathy, but strong evidence with respect to clinical efficacy is lacking. In a randomized, placebo-controlled trial comparing PRP with saline injection, De Vos and colleagues[93] demonstrated statistically significant improvement compared with baseline for pain and level of activity, based on Victorian Institute of Sports Assessment Score A. Sanchez and colleagues[94] looked at the ability of platelet-rich fibrin to enhance healing of surgically repaired Achilles tendon ruptures, demonstrating improved ankle motion, and faster return to gentle running and sport. Moreover, subjects treated with platelet-rich fibrin returned to preinjury activity levels at a mean interval of 14 weeks, an average of 8 weeks earlier than controls.

Stem Cell Therapies

Stem cell theory

MSCs, also called mesenchymal stromal cells, are adult stem cells that are multipotent and located throughout the body (**Fig. 3**). They are multipotent in that they self-renew for long periods of time and differentiate into specialized cells with specific functions, but are limited in ability to differentiate.[95] The exact regenerative mechanism of MSCs role remains unclear; however, it is believed that a primary purpose of MSCs is to replace lost or damaged cells and tissues within their local environment.

Definition

Adult MSCs are derived from perivascular cells called pericytes. Pericytes can dissociate from the basal lamina of a blood vessel becoming exposed to the chemotactic environment of the surrounding tissue and transform into an MSC.[96] The Mesenchymal and Tissue Stem Cell Committee of the International Society for Cellular Therapy proposed a more formal definition that characterizes MSCs as cells with a thin and

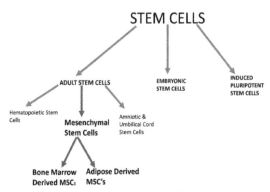

Fig. 3. Stem cell lineage. MSCs, mesenchymal stems cells. *Courtesy of* Prathap Jayaram, MD, Baylor College of Medicine, University of Texas Health Science Center, Houston, TX.

elongated morphology that can express specific surface markers and can adhere to plastic. They must also be antiinflammatory, antiapoptotic, antifibrotic, and possess immunomodulatory effects. The criteria further defines an MSC to have ability to self-replicate and differentiate into multiple cell types of mesenchymal origin.[97]

Sources

There are multiple sources of MSCs; bone marrow and adipose tissues are the current sources used in injectable orthopedic practice. The posterior superior iliac spine is the most commonly accessed landmark for bone marrow aspiration. Bone marrow aspiration is also known as bone marrow concentrate (BMC). This source provides cells containing MSCs, hematopoietic stem cells, endothelial progenitor cells, plasma, and a variety of soluble bioactive substances. Bone marrow cells can be further characterized into nucleated and nonnucleated cells. White blood cells and their precursors account for most of the nucleated cell fraction with red blood cells and megakaryocytes accounting for a smaller ratio of nucleated cells. Bone marrow MSCs (BMSCs) and hematopoietic stem cells account for an even smaller portion of nucleated cells averaging 1 in 10,000 to 1 in 50,000 of total nucleated cells. It has also been demonstrated that BMSCs viability and number are reduced by age and disease.[98] Adipose-derived MSCs are isolated from the stromal vascular fraction of homogenized adipose tissue. Adipose-derived MSCs, like BMSCs, are derived from pericytes. Compared with BMSCs, adipose-derived MSCs have a higher density per unit volume of tissue and able to proliferate in culture more quickly.[99,100] Despite these differences, there is no current evidence from clinical trials comparing adipose-derived MSCs and BMSCs for musculoskeletal injury.

Another potential regenerative injectable that has fallen out of favor clinically are amniotic tissue injections. Amniotic membrane–based products have various therapeutic applications in the foot and ankle, including the treatment of chronic wounds, fasciitis, and tendonitis. Although it is true that amniotic fluid does contain an abundant source of stem cells, the US Food and Drug Administration has only approved a form of amniotic tissue that after processing does not contain any live cells also known as dehydrated human amnion or chorion membrane.[101]

Clinical applications

Bone marrow concentrate injectables There has been an increase in clinical usefulness of using BMC injection treatment for articular cartilage defects, a common pathology affecting the elderly. Goldring and colleagues[102] demonstrated benefit of this strategy at 24 weeks after percutaneous injection into the affected knee joint, showing a significant increase in cartilage and meniscus volume on MRI. Patients also attained increase range of motion and decreased pain scores. In a recent multicenter analysis of 2372 patients who underwent stem cell injections with a follow-up of 2.2 years, a total of 325 adverse events were reported.[1] There were 7 cases of neoplasm, lower rate than in the general population with lowest rate of adverse events observed in patients receiving BMC alone, compared with BMC plus adipose and cultured cells. Sampson and colleagues[103] have reported preliminary data that was targeted cartilage defects. They showed favorable outcomes in 125 patients receiving hip, knee, shoulder, ankle, or cervical zygapophyseal joint BMC injections. There was a 71% reduction in overall pain at a median follow-up of 148 days after injection in patients. Knee injections had the greatest improvement in pain scores compared with the other joints. Satisfaction with the procedure was reported by 92% of patients, and 95% would recommend the procedure to a friend.[103,104] These studies do support the safety profile of autologous BMC therapy for articular cartilage defects, with some evidence to suggest clinical efficacy.

Although there are numerous preclinical studies on MSC therapy in spine pathology, there are few clinical studies that have examined its efficacy. Pettine and colleagues[105] examined 26 patients (11 male, 15 female, aged 18–61 years, 13 single level, 13 two level) with chronic discogenic low back pain who received BMC injections into the disc. They were able to demonstrate beneficial effects with no disc worsening on MRI, and 21 of 24 avoided surgery for 2 years with improvements in functional outcomes and pain. There are 3 other studies with smaller numbers that demonstrate strong safety profiles and have shown beneficial subjective outcomes.[106–108]

As mentioned, tendinopathy is highly prevalent in the elderly. Rotator cuff tendinopathy in particular has a significant impact on upper extremity function. Hernigou and colleagues[109] examined 90 patients 10 years after routine arthroscopy, comparing those who did and di not receive BMC injections, and found 87% of patients had intact rotator cuffs compared with 44% in the control group, suggesting that MSCs here could have enhanced recovery and/or preventing further tendon degradation.

BMC therapy has shown an excellent safety profile in current applications to orthopedic injuries and there continues to be evidence to support this; however, the challenge of understanding the regenerative mechanisms at play is still not understood fully. Now that it has been established that BMC therapy is safe, more precision based studies that incorporate dosing profiles and standardizing pathology need to be done to better delineate regenerative mechanisms. Although long-term follow-up is essential, it is equally important to standardize MSC treatments to evaluate their outcomes more critically.

Adipose-derived concentrate injectables Adipose-derived MSCs have also been used in clinical practice with a good safety profile. Koh and Choi[108] performed MSC injections derived from adipose with arthroscopic lavage in elderly patients with knee OA. At the 2-year follow-up, 14 of the 16 patients showed improved or maintained cartilage.[108] Subjective functional outcome scores, the Knee Injury Osteoarthritis Outcome, visual analog scale, and Lysholm scores also improved with statistical significance. In a smaller study of 18 patients with intraarticular knee cartilage defects, Jo and colleagues were able to show decrease in cartilage defect size, improved knee function and decreased pain after injection of adipose-derived MSCs.[109] Whereas adipose-derived MSCs have started to make more of a presence in injectable musculoskeletal strategies, more comprehensive studies need to be done to better understand the regenerative mechanisms.

Clinical indications, research, and future directions Exercise and activity in general are considered to be beneficial to health throughout life. As one ages, there are changes to the musculoskeletal system that are the result of attrition, overuse, and accumulated trauma. As a result, there is a cost to being active that is more prevalent and substantial in the older adult than in the younger adult. Musculoskeletal care will play a pivotal and continued role in the management of these conditions in the aging and active geriatric adults. There are promising therapies and emerging therapies that can help to manage and perhaps even reverse some of these changes. The use of tenotomy for tendinopathy has been demonstrated to be effective. Combining this treatment with biologic therapies such as PRP and prolotherapy may lead to more regenerative effects in tendinopathy. Stem cell treatment, although still not fully understood, is promising for tendinopathy and OA. Additional regenerative therapies, such as lipoaspirate and amniotic tissue–derived injectants with and without hyaluronic acid hold promise, and are now approved by the US Food and Drug Administration, but still poorly understood and lacking substantial evidence. Research should be focused on structural and physiologic effects of regenerative treatments and also in the clinical outcomes measured against conventional therapy.

REFERENCES

1. Malanga G, Abdelshahed D, Jayaram P. Orthobiologic interventions using ultrasound guidance. Phys Med Rehabil Clin N Am 2016;27(3):717–31.
2. Khan KM, Cook JL, Bonar F. Histopathology of common tendinopathies: update and implications for clinical management. Sports Med 1999;27:393–408.
3. Narici MV, Maffulli N, Maganaris CN. Ageing of human muscles and tendons. Disabil Rehabil 2008;30:1548–54.
4. Van der Windt DA, Koes BW, de Jong BA, et al. Shoulder disorders in general practice: incidence, patient characteristics, and management. Ann Rheum Dis 1995;54(12):959–64.
5. Milgrom C, Schaffler M, Gilbert S. Rotator-cuff changes in asymptomatic adults. The effect of age, hand dominance and gender. J Bone Joint Surg Br 1995;77: 296–8.
6. Riley GP, Harrall RL, Constant CR, et al. Glycosaminoglycans of human rotator cuff tendons: changes with age and in chronic rotator cuff tendinitis. Ann Rheum Dis 1994;53:367–76.
7. Rudzki JR, Adler RS, Warren RF. Contrast-enhanced ultrasound characterization of the vascularity of the rotator cuff tendon: age- and activity-related changes in the intact asymptomatic rotator cuff. J Shoulder Elbow Surg 2008;17(1 Suppl): 96S–100S.
8. Brinks A, van Rijn RM, Willemsen SP, et al. Corticosteroid injections for greater trochanteric pain syndrome: a randomized controlled trial in primary care. Ann Fam Med 2011;9(3):226–34.
9. Cohen SP, Strassels SA, Foster L, et al. Comparison of fluoroscopically guided and blind corticosteroid injections for greater trochanteric pain syndrome: multicentre randomized controlled trial. BMJ 2009;338:b1088.

10. Furia JP, Rompe JD, Maffulli N. Low-energy extracorporeal shock wave therapy as a treatment for greater trochanteric pain syndrome. Am J Sports Med 2009; 37(9):1806–13.

11. Labrosse JM, Cardinal E, Leduc BE, et al. Effectiveness of ultrasound-guided corticosteroid injection for the treatment of gluteus medias tendinopathy. Am J Roentgenol 2010;194(1):202–6.

12. Fearon AM, Cook JL, Scarvell JM, et al. Greater trochanteric pain syndrome negatively affects work, physical activity and quality of life: a case control study. J Arthroplasty 2014;29(2):383–6.

13. Alvarez-Nemegyei J, Canoso JJ. Evidence-based soft tissue rheumatology: III. Trochanteric bursitis. J Clin Rheumatol 2004;10(3):123–4.

14. Segal NA, Felson DT, Torner JC, et al. Greater trochanteric pain syndrome: epidemiology and associated factors. Arch Phys Med Rehabil 2007;88(8): 988–92.

15. Albers S, Zwerver J, Van den Akker-Scheek I. Incidence and prevalence of lower extremity tendinopathy in the general population. Br J Sports Med 2014; 48(Suppl 2):A5.

16. Clancy WG. Runners' injuries: part two. Evaluation and treatment of specific injuries. Am J Sports Med 1980;8(4):287–9.

17. Sutter R, Kalberer F, Binkert CA, et al. Abductor tendon tears are associated with hypertrophy of the tensor fasciae lata muscle. Skeletal Radiol 2013;42(5): 627–33.

18. Pfirrmann CW, Notzli HP, Dora C, et al. Abductor tendons and muscles assessed at MR imaging after total hip arthroplasty in asymptomatic and symptomatic patients. Radiology 2005;235(3):969–76.

19. Birnbaum K, Prescher A, Niethard FU. Hip centralizing forces of the iliotibial tract within various femoral neck angles. J Pediatr Orthop B 2010;19(2):140–9.

20. Kountouris A, Cook J. Rehabilitation of Achilles and patellar tendinopathies. Best Pract Res Clin Rheumatol 2007;21(2):295–316.

21. Peers KH, Lysens RJ. Patellar tendinopathy in athletes: current diagnostic and therapeutic recommendations. Sports Med 2005;35(1):71–87.

22. Grau S, Maiwald C, Krauss I, et al. What are causes and treatment strategies for patellar-tendinopathy in female runners? J Biomech 2008;41(9):2042–6.

23. Couppe C, Hansen P, Kongsgaard M, et al. Mechanical properties and collagen cross-linking of the patellar tendon in old and young men. J Appl Physiol 2009; 107:880–6.

24. Carroll CC, Dickinson JM, Haus JM, et al. Influence of aging on the in vivo properties of human patellar tendon. J Appl Physiol 2008;105:1907–15.

25. Garcia C, Martin RL, Houck J, et al. Achilles pain, stiffness, and muscle power deficits: Achilles tendinitis. Clinical practice guidelines linked to the international classification of functioning, disability, and health from the orthopedic section of the American Physical Therapy Association. J Orthop Sports Phys Ther 2010; 40(9):A1–26.

26. Turan A, Teber MA, Yakut ZI, et al. Sonoelastographic assessment of the age-related changes of the Achilles tendon. J Med Ultrason 2015;17(1):58–61.

27. Evans CH, Ghivizzani SC, Smith P, et al. Using gene therapy to protect and restore cartilage. Clin Orthop Relat Res 2000;(379 Suppl):S214–9.

28. Brown TD, Johnston RC, Saltzman CL, et al. Posttraumatic osteoarthritis: a first estimate of incidence, prevalence, and burden of disease. J Orthop Trauma 2006;20(10):739–44.

29. Hartvigsen J, Frederiksen H, Christensen K. Back and neck pain in seniors-prevalence and impact. Eur Spine J 2006;15:802–6.
30. Boake C, McCauley SR, Levin HS, et al. Diagnostic criteria for postconcussional syndrome after mild to moderate traumatic brain injury. J Neuropsychiatry Clin Neurosci 2005;17:350–6.
31. Deyo RA, Loeser JD, Bigos SJ. Herniated lumbar intervertebral disk. Ann Intern Med 1990;112(8):598–603.
32. Spangfort EV. The lumbar disc herniation. A computer aided analysis of 2504 operations. Acta Orthop Scand Suppl 1972;142:1–95.
33. Anderson G. Epidemiology of spinal disorders. In: Frymoyer JW, Ducker TB, Hadler NM, et al, editors. The adult spine: principles and practice. New York: Raven Press; 1997. p. 93–141.
34. Pérez-Prieto D, Lozano-Álvarez C, Saló G, et al. Should age be a contraindication for degenerative lumbar surgery? Eur Spine J 2014;23:1007–12.
35. Siebert E, Pruss H, Klingebiel R, et al. Lumbar spinal stenosis: syndrome, diagnostics and treatment. Nat Rev Neurosci 2009;5(7):392–403.
36. Bodack MP, Monteiro M. Therapeutic exercise in the treatment of patient with lumbar spinal stenosis. Clin Orthop Relat Res 2001;384:144–52.
37. Balazs EA, Watson D, Duff IF, et al. Hyaluronic acid in synovial fluid: I. molecular parameters of hyaluronic acid in normal and arthritis human fluids. Arthritis Rheum 1967;10:357–76.
38. Strauss EJ, Hart JA, Miller MD, et al. Hyaluronic acid viscosupplementation and osteoarthritis: current uses and future directions. Am J Sports Med 2009;37: 1636–44.
39. Conrozier T, Chevalier X. Long-term experience with hylan GF-20 in the treatment of knee osteoarthritis. Expert Opin Pharmacother 2008;9:1797–804.
40. Balazs EA, Denlinger JL. Viscosupplementation: a new concept in the treatment of osteoarthritis. J Rheumatol Suppl 1993;39:3–9.
41. Ghosh P, Guidolin D. Potential mechanism of action of intra-articular hyaluronan therapy in osteoarthritis: are the effects molecular weight dependent? Semin Arthritis Rheum 2002;32:10–37.
42. Wang CT, Lin J, Chang CJ, et al. Therapeutic effects of hyaluronic acid on osteoarthritis of the knee: a meta-analysis of randomized controlled trials. J Bone Joint Surg Am 2004;86-A:538–45.
43. Taylor MA, Norman TL, Clovis NB, et al. The response of rabbit patellar tendon after autologous blood injection. Med Sci Sports Exerc 2002;34(1):70–3.
44. Mattie R, Wong J, McCormick Z, et al. Percutaneous needle tenotomy of lateral epicondylitis: a systemic review of the literature. PM R 2016;9(6):603–11.
45. Jacobson JA, Rubin J, Yablon CM, et al. Ultrasound-guided fenestration of tendons about the hip and pelvis: clinical outcomes. J Ultrasound Med 2015;34: 2029–35.
46. Housner JA, Jacobson JA, Misko R. Sonographically guided percutaneous needle tenotomy for the treatment of chronic tendinosis. J Ultrasound Med 2009;28: 1187–92.
47. McShane JM, Shah VN, Nazarian LN. Sonographically guided percutaneous needle tenotomy for treatment of common extensor tendinosis in the elbow: is a corticosteroid necessary? J Ultrasound Med 2008;27:1137–44.
48. Dragoo JL, Wasterlain A, Braun HJ, et al. Platelet rich plasma as a treatment for patellar tendinopathy; a double blind, randomized controlled trial. Am J Sports Med 2014;42:610–8.

49. Alfredson H, Ohberg L. Neovascularization in chronic painful patellar tendinosis: promising results after sclerosing neovessels outside the tendon challenge the for surgery. Knee Surg Sports Traumatol Arthrosc 2005;13:74–80.

50. Barnes DE, Beckley JM, Smith J. Percutaneous ultrasonic tenotomy for chronic elbow tendinosis: a prospective study. J Shoulder Elbow Surg 2015;24:67–73.

51. Reeves KD. Technique of prolotherapy. In: Lennard TA, editor. Physiatric procedures in clinical practice. Philadelphia: Hanley & Belfus; 1995. p. 57–70.

52. Hackett GS. Prolotherapy in whiplash and low back pain. Postgrad Med 1960; 27:214–9.

53. Hackett GS. Ligament and tendon relaxation treated by prolotherapy. 3rd edition. Springfield (IL): Charles C Thomas; 1956.

54. Banks A. A rationale for prolotherapy. J Orthop Med (UK) 1991;13(3):54–9.

55. Kim SR, Stitik TP, Foye PM. Critical review of prolotherapy for osteoarthritis, low back pain and other musculoskeletal conditions; a physiatric perspective. Am J Phys Med Rehabil 2004;83:379–89.

56. Hirschberg GG, Froetscher L, Naiem F. Iliolumbar syndrome as a common cause of low back pain: diagnosis and prognosis. Arch Phys Med Rehabil 1979;60:516–9.

57. Hirschberg GG, Williams KA, Byrd JG. Medical management of iliocostal pain. Geriatrics 1992;47:62–8.

58. Klein RG, Dorman TA, Johnson CE. Proliferant injections for low back pain: histologic changes of injected ligaments and objective measurements of lumbar spine mobility before and after treatment. J Neurol Orthop Med Surg 1989;10: 141–4.

59. Miller MR, Matthews RS, Reeves KD. Treatment of painful advanced internal lumbar disc derangement with intradiscal injection of hyperosmolar dextrose. Pain Physician 2006;9:115–21.

60. Park YS, Lim SW, Lee IH, et al. Intra-articular injection of a nutritive mixture solution protects articular cartilage from osteoarthritic progression induced by anterior cruciate ligament transection in mature rabbits: a randomized controlled trial. Arthritis Res Ther 2007;9:R8.

61. Reeves KD. A randomized prospective double blind placebo controlled study of dextrose prolotherapy for knee osteoarthritis with or without ACL laxity. Altern Ther Health Med 2000;6:68–80.

62. Dumais R, Benoit C. Effect of regenerative injection therapy on function and pain in patients with knee osteoarthritis: a randomized crossover study. Pain Med 2012;13(8):990–9.

63. Rabago D, Patterson JJ, Mundt M, et al. Dextrose prolotherapy for knee osteoarthritis: a randomized controlled trial. Ann Fam Med 2013;11:229–37.

64. Topol GA, Podesta LA, Reeves KD, et al. Chondrogenic effect of intra-articular hypertonic-dextrose (prolotherapy) in severe knee osteoarthritis. PM R 2016;8: 1072–82.

65. Reeves KD, Hassanein K. Randomized prospective placebo controlled double blind study of dextrose prolotherapy for osteoarthritic thumbs and finger. J Altern Complement Med 2000;6(4):311–20.

66. Rabago D, Best TM, Zgierska AE, et al. A systematic review of four injection therapies for lateral epicondylosis: prolotherapy, polidocinol, whole blood and platelet rich plasma. Br J Sports Med 2009;43:471–81.

67. Ryan M, Wong A, Rabago D, et al. Ultrasound-guided injections of hyperosmolar dextrose for overuse patellar tendinopathy: a pilot study. Br J Sports Med 2011;45:972–7.

68. Maxwell NJ, Ryan MB, Taunton JE, et al. Sonographically guided intratendinous injection of hyperosmolar dextrose to treat chronic tendinosis of the Achilles tendon: a pilot study. Am J Roentgenol 2007;189:W215-20.

69. Ryan M, Wong A, Taunton J. Favorable outcomes after sonographically guided intratendinous injection of hyperosmolar dextrose for chronic insertional and midportion Achilles tendinosis. Am J Roentgenol 2010;194:1047-53.

70. Ryan MB, Wong AD, Gillies JH, et al. Sonographically guided intratendinous injections of hyperosmolar dextrose/lidocaine: a pilot study for the treatment of chronic plantar fasciitis. Br J Sports Med 2009;43:303-6.

71. Kim E, Lee JH. Autologous platelet rich plasma versus dextrose prolotherapy for the treatment of chronic recalcitrant plantar fasciitis. PM R 2014;6:152-8.

72. Best LM, Best TM. Prolotherapy: a clinical review of its role in treating chronic musculoskeletal pain. PM R 2011;3:S78-81.

73. Rabago D, Best TM, Beamsley M, et al. A systematic review of prolotherapy for chronic musculoskeletal pain. Clin J Sport Med 2005;15(5):376-80.

74. Khan M, Bedi A. Cochrane in CORR: platelet-rich therapies for musculoskeletal soft tissue injuries. Clin Orthop Relat Res 2015;473(7):2207-13.

75. Mishra A, Harmon K, Woodall J, et al. Sports medicine applications of platelet rich plasma. Curr Pharm Biotechnol 2012;13:1185-95.

76. Dohan Ehrenfest DM, Rasmusson L, Albrektsson T. Classification of platelet concentrates, from pure platelet-rich plasma (PPRP) to leucocyte- and platelet-rich fibrin (L-PRF). Trends Biotechnol 2009;27:158-67.

77. Dohan Ehrenfest DM, Bielecki T, Mishra A, et al. In search of a consensus terminology in the field of platelet concentrates for surgical use: platelet-rich plasma (PRP), platelet-rich fibrin (PRF), fibrin glue polymerization and leukocytes. Curr Pharm Biotechnol 2012;13:1131-7.

78. DeLong JM, Russell RP, Mazzocca AD. Platelet-rich plasma: the PAW classification system. Arthroscopy 2012;28:998-1009.

79. Mautner K, Malanga GA, Smith J, et al. A call for a standard classification system for future biologic research: the rationale for new PRP nomenclature. PM R 2015;7(4 Suppl):S53-9.

80. Mazzocca AD, McCarthy MB, Chowaniec DM, et al. Platelet-rich plasma differs according to preparation method and human variability. J Bone Joint Surg Am 2012;94(4):308-16.

81. Malanga G, Nakamura R. The role of regenerative medicine in the treatment of sports injuries. Phys Med Rehabil Clin N Am 2014;25(4):881-95.

82. Coombes BK, Bisset L, Vicenzino B. Efficacy and safety of corticosteroid injections and other injections for management of tendinopathy: a systematic review of randomized controlled trials. Lancet 2010;376:1751-67.

83. Weber SC, Kauffman NJ, Parise C, et al. Platelet-rich plasma matrix in the management of arthroscopic repair of the rotator cuff. Am J Sports Med 2012;41:263-70.

84. Jo CH, Kim JE, Yoon KS, et al. Does platelet-rich plasma accelerate recovery after rotator cuff repair? Am J Sports Med 2011;39:2082-90.

85. Bergeson AG, Tashjian RZ, Greis PE, et al. Effects of platelet-rich fibrin matrix on repair integrity of at-risk rotator cuff tears. Am J Sports Med 2012;40:286-93.

86. Kesikburun S, Tan AK, Yilmaz B, et al. Platelet-rich plasma injections in the treatment of chronic rotator cuff tendinopathy: a randomized controlled trial with 1-year follow-up. Am J Sports Med 2013;41:2609-16.

87. Rha DW, Park GY, Kim YK, et al. Comparison of the therapeutic effects of ultrasound-guided platelet-rich plasma injection and dry needling in rotator cuff disease: a randomized controlled trial. Clin Rehabil 2012;27:113–22.
88. Lee JJ, Harrison JR, Boachie-Adjei K, et al. Platelet-rich plasma injections with needle tenotomy for gluteus medius tendinopathy. Orthop J Sports Med 2016; 4(11). 2325967116671692.
89. Kon E, Filardo G, Delcogliano M, et al. Platelet-rich plasma: new clinical application a pilot study for treatment of jumper's knee. Injury 2009;40:598–603.
90. James SL, Ali K, Pocock C, et al. Ultrasound guided dry needling and autologous blood injection for patellar tendinosis. Br J Sports Med 2007;41:518–22.
91. Everhart JS, Cole D, Sojka JH, et al. Treatment options for patellar tendinopathy: a systematic review. Arthroscopy 2017;33(4):861–72.
92. de Vos RJ, Weir A, van Schie HT, et al. Platelet-rich plasma injection for chronic Achilles tendinopathy: a randomized controlled trial. JAMA 2010;303:144–9.
93. Sanchez M, Anitua E, Azofra J, et al. Comparison of surgically repaired Achilles tendon tears using platelet-rich fibrin matrices. Am J Sports Med 2007;35: 245–51.
94. Caplan AI. All MSCs are pericytes? Cell Stem Cell 2008;3(3):229–30.
95. Dominici M, Le Blanc K, Mueller I, et al. Minimal criteria for defining multipotent mesenchymal stromal cells. The International Society for Cellular Therapy position statement. Cytotherapy 2006;8(4):315–7.
96. Toraño EG, Bayón GF, del Real Á, et al. Age-associated hydroxymethylation in human bone-marrow mesenchymal stem cells. J Transl Med 2016;14:207.
97. Kern S, Eichler H, Stoeve J, et al. Comparative analysis of mesenchymal stem cells from bone marrow, umbilical cord blood, or adipose tissue. Stem Cells 2006;24:1294–301.
98. Izadpanah R, Trygg C, Patel B, et al. Biologic properties of mesenchymal stem cells derived from bone marrow and adipose tissue. J Cell Biochem 2006;99: 1285–97.
99. Zelen C, Snyder R, Serena T, et al. The use of human amnion/chorion membrane in the clinical setting for lower extremity repair: a review. Clin Podiatr Med Surg 2015;32(1):135–46.
100. Goldring MB. The role of the chondrocyte in osteoarthritis. Arthritis Rheum 2000; 43:1916–26.
101. Centeno CJ, Al-Sayegh H, Freeman MD, et al. A multi-center analysis of adverse events among two thousand, three hundred and seventy two adult patients undergoing adult autologous stem cell therapy for orthopaedic conditions. Int Orthop 2016;40:1755.
102. Sampson S, Botto-Van Bemden A, Aufiero D. Stem cell therapies for treatment of cartilage and bone disorders: osteoarthritis, avascular necrosis and non-union fractures. PM R 2015;7(4):S26–32.
103. Pettine K, Suzuki R, Sand T, et al. Treatment of discogenic back pain with autologous bone marrow concentrate injection with minimum two year follow-up. Int Orthop 2016;40:135.
104. Mochida J, Sakai D, Nakamura Y, et al. Intervertebral disc repair with activated nucleus pulposus cell transplantation: a three-year, prospective clinical study of its safety. Eur Cell Mater 2015;29:202–12.
105. Orozco L, Soler R, Morera C, et al. Intervertebral disc repair by autologous mesenchymal bone marrow cells: a pilot study. Transplantation 2011;92(7): 822–8.

106. Yoshikawa T, Ueda Y, Miyazaki K, et al. Disc regeneration therapy using marrow mesenchymal cell transplantation: a report of two case studies. Spine 2010; 35(11):E475–80.
107. Hernigou P, Flouzat Lachaniette CH, Delambre J, et al. Biologic augmentation of rotator cuff repair with mesenchymal stem cells during arthroscopy improves healing and prevents further tears: a case-controlled study. Int Orthop 2014; 38(9):1811–8.
108. Koh YG, Choi YJ. Infrapatellar fat pad-derived mesenchymal stem cell therapy for knee osteoarthritis. Knee 2012;19:902–7.
109. Jo CH, Lee YG, Shin WH, et al. Intra-articular injection of mesenchymal stem cells for the treatment of osteoarthritis of the knee: a proof-of-concept clinical trial. Stem Cells 2014;32(5):1254–66.

Clinical Considerations for the Use Lower Extremity Arthroplasty in the Elderly

Antonio Otero-López, MD*, David Beaton-Comulada, MD

KEYWORDS

- Total knee arthroplasty • Total hip arthroplasty • Elderly • Osteoarthritis
- Rehabilitation

KEY POINTS

- There is an increase in the aging population, which has led to a surge of cases of osteoarthritis (OA) and demand for lower extremity arthroplasty.
- Elderly patients have special needs and medical comorbidities that must be assessed during planning. Perioperative management is key to reduce complications and improve outcomes.
- Advances in the field of arthroplasty have made this surgery a viable option for elderly patients with symptomatic OA.
- Return to previous physical activity and excellent clinical outcomes can be obtained in elderly patients with proper surgical management, postoperative care, and collaboration with other specialties.

INTRODUCTION

There is an increase in the aging population. Demographic studies have shown that from 2000 to 2010, the age group older than 65 year old in the United States increased at a faster rate than the total population (15.1% and 9.7%, respectively).[1] As a result, there has been an increase in the prevalence of diseases associated with advanced age, such as osteoarthritis (OA) and osteoporosis.[2] The estimated lifetime risk of developing hip and knee OA is 25% and 45%, respectively.[3,4] The most common indication for total joint arthroplasty is OA of the hip or knee, one of the most common causes of mobility impairment in the elderly.[5,6] The reported lifetime risk of undergoing a total knee arthroplasty (TKA) or total hip arthroplasty (THA) owing to end-stage OA is

Disclosure Statement: The authors have nothing to disclose.
Department of Orthopaedic Surgery, School of Medicine, University of Puerto Rico, University of Puerto Rico Medical Sciences Campus, PO Box 365067, San Juan, PR 00936-5067, USA
* Corresponding author.
E-mail address: Antonio.otero3@upr.edu

Phys Med Rehabil Clin N Am 28 (2017) 795–810
http://dx.doi.org/10.1016/j.pmr.2017.06.011
1047-9651/17/Published by Elsevier Inc.
pmr.theclinics.com

10% to 11% and 6% to 7%, respectively.[7] This is mainly due to TKA and THA providing pain relief and improvement in quality of life, with greater than 90% prosthesis survival at 10 years.[8] This upward trend of OA patients is expected continue and boost the demand for total joint arthroplasty. Kurtz and colleagues[9] estimated that by 2030 the demand for THA will increase by 174% and TKA by 673%. This article aims to provide an up-to-date literature review on current treatment options and expectations when considering lower extremity arthroplasty in the elderly patient.

Patient Evaluation

Pertinent medical history toward the chief complaint, past medical history, and family history are essential to making a proper diagnosis. Adequate physical examination (PE) of the lower extremity entails inspection, palpation, range of motion, muscle testing, motor test, and sensory evaluation of the ipsilateral and contralateral extremity. OA patients tend to present with clinical symptoms of stiffness, pain, and deformity. The pain has been described as a deep, poorly localized, aching, exacerbated by activity, and relieved with rest.[10] PE findings include tenderness to palpation, limited range of motion, and joint crepitus caused by softening of the articular cartilage.[10] OA of the hip typically presents with a gradual onset of anterior thigh or groin pain, with the earliest PE finding being decreased internal rotation of the hip. Knee OA typically presents with findings of deep pain, stiffness, swelling, and laxity owing to joint erosion. The PE findings of knee OA can be angular deformity (varus or valgus), mild effusion, and crepitus around the patellofemoral joint.[11]

Imaging studies are fundamental to the evaluation of joint OA. Weight-bearing radiographs of both knees in full extension are used to evaluate the knee. Additional knee views may be ordered, such as a posteroanterior view in 30° of knee flexion and the patellar sunrise view to evaluate the patellofemoral joint. Hip views are a low-profile anteroposterior view and lateral views of the pelvis and hip. Imaging studies serve the dual purposes of evaluating disease progression and preoperative planning in the surgical patient.[12,13] Last, it is important to always evaluate for common differential diagnosis in the assessment of the joint OA, such as infection, trauma, inflammatory disease, and malignancy.

Pharmacologic Treatment

From 2013 to 2015, 49.6% of people 65 years of age or older in the United States reported doctor-diagnosed arthritis.[14] The goals of management in OA are pain control, restoration or maintenance of an active lifestyle and improvement in joint function. In 2013, the American Academy of Orthopaedic Surgeons (AAOS) developed clinical guidelines for the management of OA of the knee (**Table 1**).[15] However, it was made clear that these guidelines do not supersede clinical experience.

Nonsteroidal antiinflammatory drugs

Nonsteroidal antiinflammatory drugs (NSAIDs) remain one of the first line treatment options in the management of OA. This preferences is due to multiple studies showing improvement of symptoms with its use.[16,17] The NSAIDs mechanism of action is through inhibition of the inflammatory response by blocking prostaglandins production via the inhibition of the cyclooxygenase enzyme.[18] It also exhibits both analgesic and antipyretic properties. Side effects may include minor dyspepsia, heart problems, and gastrointestinal hemorrhage. With advancing age, there is an increased risk of gastrointestinal hemorrhage when using NSAIDs[19]; careful evaluation of patient risk factors must be made when prescribing these medications.

Table 1	
Summary of AAOS current guidelines	
Treatment Modality	**Recommendation**
Nonsteroidal antiinflammatory drugs	Strong recommendation in favor of their use
Corticosteroid injections	Inconclusive
Opioids	Inconclusive
Viscosupplementation	Strong recommendation against its use
Glucosamine-chondroitin sulfate	Strong recommendation against its use
Platelet-rich plasma protein	Inconclusive
Rehabilitation, education, and wellness activity	Strong recommendation in favor of its use
Weight loss	Inconclusive

Data from Brown GA. AAOS Clinical Practice Guideline: Treatment of Osteoarthritis of the Knee: Evidence-Based Guideline, 2nd Edition. Journal of the American Academy of Orthopaedic Surgeons 2013;21(9):577–9.

Corticosteroid injections
Corticosteroid injections are frequently used in the management of joint OA for pain reduction. The most common route is through an intraarticular injection. This is done to both localize its effect and reduce systemic spread.[20] Complications are minimal, with transient injection site pain being the most frequent. An additional concern is the chondrotoxic effect of corticosteroids on cartilage, because recent animal studies show a dose-dependent toxicity with the use of corticosteroids.[21] However, the effects of such findings remain inconclusive and further studies are needed on this subject.[15]

Opioids
Opioids are another medication for pain management in OA. Their mechanism of action is through interaction with mu, delta, or kappa opioid receptors.[18] In elderly patients, an approximate 6% to 9% of the population use opioids for chronic pain management.[22] It was most commonly used in females diagnosed with arthritis and depression.[23] Reported side effect include drowsiness, respiratory depression, urinary retention, nausea, vomiting, and constipation.[22] They should be avoided in elderly patients because they may cause an increase risk in confusion, sedation, and delirium.[22] A recent study by Ben-Ari and colleagues[24] demonstrated that long-term opioid use before TKA was associated with an increased risk of knee revision during the first year after TKA.

Viscosupplementation
Viscosupplementation is a therapeutic modality consisting of a viscoelastic solution injected into the intraarticular space of a joint. It functions to restore the rheological properties of the synovial fluid and improve joint function. Side effects are minor but may include harm to the soft tissue components when injecting the substance. Jevsevar and colleagues[25] through a systematic review demonstrated no clinical improvement when using viscosupplementation. Still, the current recommendation has been questioned and recent systematic reviews have shown favorable outcomes when using viscosupplementation in knee OA.[26,27]

Glucosamine-chondroitin sulfate
Glucosamine is a naturally occurring aminosaccharide and is one of the main components for the biosynthesis of proteoglycan, an essential component for the proper

maintenance of cartilage.[26] It is also the most frequently used supplement by OA patients with a recommended dose of 1500 mg once a day. Most studies have continued to question its efficacy for the management of OA.[28–31] However, 2 recent studies have shown favorable outcomes with the use of glucosamine sulfate for the management of knee pain. Hochberg and colleagues[32] demonstrated comparable results between celecoxib and chondroitin sulfate at 6 months of treatment as measured by pain, stiffness, and functional limitation. Rovati and colleagues[33] demonstrated that crystalline glucosamine sulfate reduced considerably the use of NSAIDs in symptomatic OA patients.

Platelet-rich plasma injections
Platelet-rich plasma (PRP) injections are intraarticular injections containing platelet-derived growth factors from autologous platelet concentration being introduced into the knee. These growth factors act in the chondrocytes to promote cartilage matrix synthesis and increased cell growth. Thus, its direct use in cartilage may suppress the inflammatory response and aid in the healing and regenerative process of cartilaginous tissue.[34] Recent metaanalyses have shown benefits with the use of PRP in the management of OA of the knee, with up to 12 months of treatment benefit.[34–36] Joshi Jubert and colleagues[34] concluded through a randomized clinical trial that in patients older than 67 years of age, 1 intraarticular injection of PRP has similar results to 1 shot of corticosteroid. However, the AAOS states inconclusive results "recommend for or against" with the use of PRP in the management of pain control in OA of the knee.[15]

Nonpharmacologic Management

Rehabilitation, education, and wellness activity
The AAOS states a strong recommendation in favor of rehabilitation, education, and wellness activity in the management of pain control in OA of the knee.[15] They observed the following: (1) exercise interventions were mostly conducted under direct supervision, most often by a physical therapist, (2) self-management interventions were led by various health care providers, (3) statistically significant improvement with the addition of strengthening exercises to a physical therapy program versus control, (4) long-term outcomes did not vary among isometric, isotonic, or isokinetic exercises and both weight-bearing and non–weight-bearing exercises were superior to control in improving physical function, and (5) aquatic therapy is an adequate alternative to land-based strengthening exercises.

Weight loss
The AAOS states a moderate recommendation in favor of weight loss in the management of pain control in OA of the knee.[15] A systematic review by Lui and colleagues[37] concluded that there are limited studies on weight loss before total joint arthroplasty, recommending further research in this topic.

Surgical Management in the Older Patient

When conservative management fails to provide pain relief and improved functionality, more invasive treatments may be considered. The most common surgical procedure for symptomatic OA is a total joint arthroplasty owing historic excellent reported outcomes and lasting results. Currently, patients undergoing THA and TKA are of older age and with an increased number of medical comorbidities.[38] These patients have special needs that must be taken into consideration during the surgical planning to minimize complications and to optimize patient functionality and outcomes.

Diabetes
Studies have consistently identified diabetes as a risk factor for postoperative complications in total joint arthroplasty.[38] The preoperative screening for hyperglycemia is hemoglobin A_{1c} (HbA_{1c}) levels and a level greater than 6.7 is associated with an increased risk of wound complications.[39,40] Still, the optimal target HbA_{1c} has not been defined, and many patients may not be able to achieve the target HbA_{1c}.[41] There is currently an emphasis on focusing more on the trend of HbA_{1c} levels rather than an exact value to predict complications.[40] Also, acute glucose monitoring via fasting glucose levels has been a new subject, with new studies coming out assessing its efficacy in predicting complications in total joint arthroplasty.[42] Meding colleagues[43] reported that, in addition to the increased risk of infection and wound complications, diabetic patients were also at an increased risk of revision surgery than nondiabetic patients (3.6% vs 0.4%).

Obesity
Obesity is another common identifiable risk factor in total joint arthroplasty surgery, with increased complications of renal failure, cardiovascular complication and postoperative infection.[44] More than one-third of adults in the United States are classified as obese and patients presenting with the diagnosis of OA are more like to obese than the general population.[45,46] Also, obesity is an independent risk factor for revision TKA and increases the risk of component malposition during surgery.[47,48] Currently there is no absolute body mass index at which patients' risk of postoperative complications significantly increase but many studies have stratified patients as having a body mass index of greater or lesser than 40 kg/m^2.[38] Analysis of subcutaneous fat tissue in the extremity and possible complications have been recently studied.[49,50] Its rationale is that not all obese patient have the same body fat distribution and this may affect surgical exposure and implant placement.

Smoking
Tobacco is one of the strongest risk factors for surgical patients, with nearly double the risk for wound complications.[38] A period of 6 to 8 weeks of smoking cessation has been associated with a decrease in postoperative complications.

Cardiovascular disease
Cardiovascular disease is a risk factor in total joint arthroplasty, with associated cardiovascular adverse events after surgery. Currently, there are no evidence-based guidelines for antiplatelet cessation in total joint arthroplasty. However, it is recommended that, if clopidogrel is stopped for surgical management, aspirin be continued and clopidogrel be restarted soon after surgery. Stopping clopidogrel 7 days before surgery may reduce the need for perioperative transfusion from 31.8% to 7.7% without increasing perioperative adverse cardiac events.[51]

Venous thromboembolism prophylaxis
Venous thromboembolism (VTE) is a possible complication after total joint arthroplasty surgery. The American College of Chest Physicians recommends one of the following agents for VTE prophylaxis: low-molecular-weight heparin (enoxaparin), vitamin K antagonists (warfarin), aspirin, factor Xa inhibitors, direct thrombin inhibitors, and portable compression devices. They also recommend VTE prophylaxis of 10 to 14 days after lower extremity arthroplasty and it may even extend for up to 35 days in selected cases.[52] In contrast, the AAOS guidelines do not have specific recommendations for VTE prophylaxis but state moderate evidence in favor of pharmacologic agents, mechanical compression devices, or both in the prevention of VTE in patients

without an increased risk for VTE beyond that of the surgery itself.[53] There is recent interest for the use of aspirin and mechanical compression devices in VTE prophylaxis, with current studies reporting various results in favor or against the use of aspirin in VTE prophylaxis.[38] Mechanical compression devices are currently recommended by the American College of Chest Physicians based on studies suggesting efficacious VTE prophylaxis using this modality, but studies remain inconclusive and further studies are required to establish their usefulness.[52]

Blood management

Lower extremity joint arthroplasty has been associated with substantial blood loss, with a reported total blood loss of 1.5 L.[54] Part of the total blood loss is the hidden blood loss, which is composed of blood loss moved to tissues or joint space, and attributable to hemolysis, with more hidden blood loss associated in TKA (49% of total blood loss) than THA (26% of total blood loss).[54] Anemia during these procedures is associated with an increased risk of postoperative cardiovascular, genitourinary, and mortality risks.[55] Therefore, blood level optimization remains a crucial component in the perioperative evaluation of arthroplasty patients. Reported anemia before surgery is 25% and postoperative anemia is approximately 51%.[56] Postoperative blood transfusion for THA have been reported to be between 37% to 53% and for TKA 46%.[57] Markers of patients requiring postoperative blood transfusion are preoperative anemia, elderly patients, multiple comorbidities, increase surgical time, and the use of postoperative anticoagulation.[57]

There are numerous protocols for the blood management in an arthroplasty, but no clear consensus on this topic. This lack is mainly due to the complexity of multiple factors such as the actual surgery, patient medical comorbidities, preoperative hemoglobin levels, and anticipated blood loss. Preoperative blood conservative strategies include preoperative screening of nutritional and hemoglobin levels with referral to a hematologist when a hemoglobin lower than 12 is reported,[58] optimization of medical comorbidities, cessation of anticoagulants or antiplatelet agents before surgery (taking into account cardiovascular risk in the patient), 4 to 6 weeks of nutritional supplements (iron, folate, vitamin B_{12}, and erythropoiesis-stimulating agents) before the planned surgery, and erythropoietin use to increase hemoglobin levels in selected patients, such as those with a high risk with allogenic transfusion. Intraoperative strategies of blood management include the use of intraoperative tourniquet, hypotensive epidural anesthesia use with extreme caution, and antifibrinolytic agents like tranexamic acid.[59,60]

Operative Techniques and Implant Selection

In the elderly population, as in the general population, pain reduction and functionality after lower extremity arthroplasty depend on accurate replacement of components and bone preparation. The current emphasis of total joint arthroplasty is on less invasive surgical approaches, aiming to protect and dissect less muscle tissue. Application of these technical considerations in patients with age-related osteoporosis can serve to improve outcomes and satisfaction.

Total knee arthroplasty

The classic approach to the knee for TKA has been an anterior skin incision combined with a medial parapatellar arthrotomy. With the renewal interest of unicompartmental knee arthroplasty, there is now an interest in minimally invasive approaches (MIA) in TKA. The goal of these approaches are to reduce soft tissue damage in TKA, such as the quadriceps muscle and extensor mechanism, improve recovery time and functional outcomes.[61] The comparison between the traditional approach and MIA remains inconclusive. Earlier studies supported MIA over the traditional approach, but poor study design and the low level of evidence in these studies have called these results in question.[62–66] Also, contemporary studies have shown no clinical advantage in the use of MIA over the traditional TKA approach.[67–70] The possible benefits of MIA have been questioned owing to documented increased risks of wound complications, surgical time, and potential loosening owing to inaccurate component placement or alignment.[61]

Simultaneous bilateral TKA has been increasing lately in patients with bilateral symptomatic knee OA. It has the advantage of including bilateral functional recovery, with only a single surgery and anesthetic use. Favorable outcomes have been reported in quality-adjusted life years, satisfaction, and quicker return to function.[71–74] However, Restrepo and colleagues[75] and Fu and colleagues[73] have reported increase risks of cardiac complications, pulmonary embolism, and death. Still, the possibility of symmetric rehabilitation has made this an attractive procedure for the elderly population, but proper patient selection must be made owing to the stated risks.

Total hip arthroplasty

The most common approach to THA is the posterior approach and its variations (posterolateral or miniposterior). It spares the abductor musculature of the hip and allows for visualization of the acetabulum and femur. Repair of the posterior capsule, external rotators, and increase in femoral prosthesis head diameter have significantly reduced the risk of dislocation after performing a posterior hip approach in THA.[76,77] It is also associated with a lower risk of lateral femoral cutaneous nerve neuropraxia, superior gluteal nerve palsy, heterotopic bone formation, abductor insufficiency, and intraoperative femoral fracture when compared with the direct anterior or lateral approach.[78] However, the posterior approach is associated with a slightly higher risk of dislocation and sciatic nerve injury when compared with the direct anterior and lateral approach to the hip.[79]

The direct anterior approach is used in 20% of THA. It is an internervous approach of the hip with an emphasis on avoiding soft tissue disruption and preservation of the basic hip anatomy.[79] Multiple randomized, controlled trials and metaanalyses comparing the anterior approach to other approaches have shown significant benefits of anterior approach in pain reduction, shorter duration of hospital stay, faster return to physical activity, and better physical well-being during the first 6 weeks to 1 year.[80–82] However, long-term results are similar at 2 years.[80] Presently, there is no clear long-term advantage between either of these approaches to the hip, because both have shown adequate results in THA.

COMPLICATIONS IN LOWER EXTREMITY ARTHROPLASTY

As with any surgical procedure, complications can arise in lower extremity arthroplasty surgery. Periprosthetic fracture risk of 2.5% to 38% and 0.4% to 4.0% have been reported in primary TKA and THA, respectively.[83,84] Johnston and colleagues[85] identified the following periprosthetic fracture risk factors in TKA surgery: osteoporosis, advanced age, female gender, malnutrition, and body mass index, an important finding, because most elderly patients present with 1 or a multiple of these associated risk factors. Also, the growing use of noncemented femoral components in THA has increased the rate of intraoperative fractures from 0.04% in cemented to approximately 5% in noncemented femoral components.[86,87] Periprosthetic joint infection (PJI) is another common cause for revision surgery. PJI risk of 1.0% to 2.3% and 0.3% to 2.2% have been reported in primary TKA and THA, respectively.[83,88] The most frequent cause for TKA revision is PJI, occurring in 25% of all revision cases.[89] There is an upward trend (1.99% in 2002 to 2.46% in 2011) in the number of cases reported to have suffered a PJI after THA.[90]

Polyethylene wear is another cause of revision surgery. Although there is a decreasing trend in revision surgery owing to associated polyethylene wear and osteolysis, they remain a common late complication of TKA surgery, with a reported 18.5% of revision surgeries performed because of them.[91–94] Instability after THA remains a challenge, with a reported incidence of 0.3% to 10.0% after primary THA and up to 28% in revision.[84] However, the use of larger femoral heads in THA have reduced the risk of dislocation and coincidentally the dislocation rate of the Medicare population undergoing THA as described by Malkani and colleagues.[95] Although complications in total joint arthroplasty can occur, it remains one of the most beneficial and impactful surgeries in medicine. Continued monitoring of complications and their solutions can further enhance patient satisfaction and functional outcome.

Pain Management and Rehabilitation

In the current multidisciplinary approach model, patient who will undergo THA are optimized before surgery and an emphasis is placed on a faster recovery.[96] This factor is especially important in the elderly, because early mobilization has been associated with better outcomes in this population. The recovery of TKA can be arduous, with anticipated knee pain during the recovery phase cited by the patient as a reason for worse outcomes.[97] Lombardi and colleagues[98] highlighted that optimization of the following factors on TKA patients can lead to improved outcomes: patient selection, patient education, pain management, regional anesthesia, intraoperative medications, postoperative medications, home medications, blood management, surgery, and postoperative care.

A multimodal approach in pain management should be used, starting with pain control before, during, and after the operation. Oral medications (nonnarcotics, NSAIDs, antiemetics) are one of the most common pain management modalities. There is a global consensus on decline usage of opioids owing to adverse effects; special attention has been placed on limiting use on the elderly owing to neurologic and respiratory side effects. The use of neuraxial or regional anesthesia produce better pain control and less adverse events when compared with general anesthesia.[99,100] Periarticular injections are also another suitable pain control option, with satisfactory results.[101,102] Peripheral nerve blocks have also shown satisfactory results, but a potential disadvantage to their use is associated muscle weakness, potentially increasing the risk of postoperative falls.[103]

Physical therapy aids both in pain control and return to functional activity after total joint arthroplasty. Patient who received physical therapy at home have demonstrated equal results as those who have physical therapy in an inpatient rehabilitation after TKA.[104,105] The surge of rapid recovery programs (discharge home after 1 to 3 days from the hospital) in THA has become the standard of care in multiple centers. Studies have shown that older patients benefit the most from these programs.[106,107]

Outcome and Lifestyle After Lower Extremity Arthroplasty in the Elderly

Total joint arthroplasty is one of the most successful surgical procedures in medicine. A recent review by Rubin and colleagues[2] demonstrated that good to excellent clinical outcomes can be obtained in the elderly population and recommends that total joint arthroplasty surgery should not be withheld in the elderly patient because it can significantly improve their quality of life. Multiple studies have shown that significant improvement can be obtained in the following areas after total joint arthroplasty surgery: pain, range of motion, and functional score.[108–110]

These procedures have been proven to be beneficial even for patients greater than 90 years of age. Reports of patients in this age group who underwent TKA showed excellent outcomes and an improvement in quality of life. Postoperative complications were mostly nonsurgical complications and related to preexistent medical conditions.[111] Brander and colleagues[112] compared collected data from 99 consecutive elective hip and knee arthroplasties in subjects 80 years of age or older (average, 83) and compared it with data from a younger otherwise matched control group. Complication rates and duration of stay in acute care facilities were not significantly different in both groups. Pain improved significantly with 98% of TKA and 100% of THA subjects reporting mild or no pain at follow-up. Function also improved; 51% of the TKA and 54% of the THA subjects were able to walk more than 5 blocks after surgery.

Although there is a clear benefit to total joint arthroplasty surgery, elderly patients have an increased risk of complications and mortality when compared with younger patients.[2] Monitoring and optimization of these risk factors can improve outcomes. Also, the comanagement of total joint arthroplasty patients has demonstrated significant improvement in outcomes and is highly recommended.[113,114]

Although studies have shown that patient undergoing total joint arthroplasty have improved functional outcomes, improvement in physical activity has been questioned. Studies have failed to show significant increases in physical activity after total joint arthroplasty surgery.[115–117] Chang and colleagues[118] evaluated the cause of patients not returning to physical activity after TKA and found that 76% of the cases the reason for inactivity was not related to the replaced knee.

A common question is when to return to athletic activities after total joint arthroplasty surgery. Currently, there are no guidelines and most recommendations are from surveys of orthopedic surgeons based on clinical experience and preference. Low-impact activities such as swimming, bowling, stationary biking, dancing, rowing, and walking are usually allowed. Downhill and cross-country skiing, weightlifting, ice skating, and Pilates are activities that may be allowed with prior experience. High-impacts sports such as racquetball, jogging, contact sports, high-impact aerobics, baseball or softball, and snowboarding should be avoided. The recommended time of return to allowable activities is 3 to 6 months after surgery.[119–121]

Another common concern is returning to drive. Previous studies recommended a waiting period of 6 weeks before driving after THA surgery. However, a recent prospective study by Hernandez and colleagues[122] demonstrated that 87% of patients could return to their baseline brake reaction time in 2 weeks and the remaining 13% at 4 weeks. They concluded that, with new techniques in THA, most patients can return to driving within the second week.

SUMMARY

The increased demand of lower extremity arthroplasty will continue to increase with the aging population. Expectations are high, because elderly patients want to remain independent and continue an active lifestyle. Continued advances in the field of arthroplasty have made arthroplasty the best option for these patients. Still, elderly patients have special needs and medical comorbidities that must be assessed during surgical planning. Perioperative management of these factors, proper surgical management, postoperative care, and collaboration with other specialists are key to reduce complications and improve outcomes.

REFERENCES

1. Ortman JM, Velkoff VA, Hogan H. An aging nation: the older population in the United States. US Census Bureau; 2014 (Report No P25-1140). Available at: http://www.census.gov/library/publications/2014/demo/p25-1140.html. Accessed April 1, 2017.
2. Rubin LE, Blood TD, Defillo-Draiby JC. Total hip and knee arthroplasty in patients older than age 80 years. J Am Acad Orthop Surg 2016;24(10):683–90.
3. Murphy LB, Helmick CG, Schwartz TA, et al. One in four people may develop symptomatic hip osteoarthritis in his or her lifetime. Osteoarthritis Cartilage 2010;18(11):1372–9.
4. Murphy L, Schwartz TA, Helmick CG, et al. Lifetime risk of symptomatic knee osteoarthritis. Arthritis Rheum 2008;59(9):1207–13.
5. Culliford DJ, Maskell J, Beard DJ, et al. Temporal trends in hip and knee replacement in the United Kingdom: 1991 to 2006. J Bone Joint Surg Br 2010;92(1):130–5.
6. Guccione AA, Felson DT, Anderson JJ, et al. The effects of specific medical conditions on the functional limitations of elders in the Framingham Study. Am J Public Health 1994;84(3):351–8.
7. Culliford DJ, Maskell J, Kiran A, et al. The lifetime risk of total hip and knee arthroplasty: results from the UK general practice research database. Osteoarthritis Cartilage 2012;20(6):519–24.
8. Segal HE, Bellamy TN. The Joint Health Benefits Delivery Program: improving access and reducing costs–successes and pitfalls. Mil Med 1988;153(8):430–1.
9. Kurtz S, Ong K, Lau E, et al. Projections of primary and revision hip and knee arthroplasty in the United States from 2005 to 2030. J Bone Joint Surg Am 2007;89(4):780–5.
10. Letha Y. Arthritis: osteoarthritis. In: April DA, Mark CH, editors. Essentials of musculoskeletal care. 5th edition. Rosemont (IL): American Academy of Orthopaedic Surgeons; 2016. p. 32–8.
11. Robert AG. Arthritis of the knee. In: April DA, Mark CH, editors. Essentials of musculoskeletal care. 5th edition. Rosemont (IL): American Academy of Orthopaedic Surgeons; 2016. p. 678–82.
12. Tanzer M, Makhdom AM. Preoperative planning in primary total knee arthroplasty. J Am Acad Orthop Surg 2016;24(4):220–30.
13. Della Valle AG, Padgett DE, Salvati EA. Preoperative planning for primary total hip arthroplasty. J Am Acad Orthop Surg 2005;13(7):455–62.
14. Barbour KE, Helmick CG, Boring M, et al. Vital signs: prevalence of doctor-diagnosed arthritis and arthritis-attributable activity limitation - United States, 2013-2015. MMWR Morb Mortal Wkly Rep 2017;66(9):246–53.
15. American Academy of Orthopaedic Surgeons. Treatment of osteoarthritis of the knee: evidence-based guideline. In: AAOS current guidelines 2013. 2017. Available at: http://www.aaos.org/research/guidelines/TreatmentofOsteoarthritisofthe KneeGuideline.pdf. Accessed March 22, 2017.
16. Gibofsky A, Williams GW, McKenna F, et al. Comparing the efficacy of cyclooxygenase 2-specific inhibitors in treating osteoarthritis: appropriate trial design considerations and results of a randomized, placebo-controlled trial. Arthritis Rheum 2003;48(11):3102–11.
17. Fleischmann R, Sheldon E, Maldonado-Cocco J, et al. Lumiracoxib is effective in the treatment of osteoarthritis of the knee: a prospective randomized 13-week study versus placebo and celecoxib. Clin Rheumatol 2006;25(1):42–53.

18. Bovill JG. Mechanisms of actions of opioids and non-steroidal anti-inflammatory drugs. Eur J Anaesthesiol Suppl 1997;15:9–15.

19. Hernandez-Diaz S, Rodriguez LA. Association between nonsteroidal anti-inflammatory drugs and upper gastrointestinal tract bleeding/perforation: an overview of epidemiologic studies published in the 1990s. Arch Intern Med 2000;160(14):2093–9.

20. Evans CH, Kraus VB, Setton LA. Progress in intra-articular therapy. Nat Rev Rheumatol 2014;10(1):11–22.

21. Wernecke C, Braun HJ, Dragoo JL. The effect of intra-articular corticosteroids on articular cartilage: a systematic review. Orthop J Sports Med 2015;3(5). 2325967115581163.

22. Naples JG, Gellad WF, Hanlon JT. The role of opioid analgesics in geriatric pain management. Clin Geriatr Med 2016;32(4):725–35.

23. Steinman MA, Komaiko KD, Fung KZ, et al. Use of opioids and other analgesics by older adults in the United States, 1999-2010. Pain Med 2015;16(2):319–27.

24. Ben-Ari A, Chansky H, Rozet I. Preoperative opioid use is associated with early revision after total knee arthroplasty: a study of male patients treated in the veterans affairs system. J Bone Joint Surg Am 2017;99(1):1–9.

25. Jevsevar D, Donnelly P, Brown GA, et al. Viscosupplementation for osteoarthritis of the knee: a systematic review of the evidence. J Bone Joint Surg Am 2015; 97(24):2047–60.

26. Percope de Andrade MA, Campos TV, Abreu ESGM. Supplementary methods in the nonsurgical treatment of osteoarthritis. Arthroscopy 2015;31(4):785–92.

27. Miller LE, Block JE. US-Approved intra-articular hyaluronic acid injections are safe and effective in patients with knee osteoarthritis: systematic review and meta-analysis of randomized, saline-controlled trials. Clin Med Insights Arthritis Musculoskelet Disord 2013;6:57–63.

28. Roman-Blas JA, Castaneda S, Sanchez-Pernaute O, et al. Combined treatment with chondroitin sulfate and glucosamine sulfate shows no superiority over placebo for reduction of joint pain and functional impairment in patients with knee osteoarthritis: a six-month multicenter, randomized, double-blind, placebo-controlled clinical trial. Arthritis Rheumatol 2017;69(1):77–85.

29. Wandel S, Juni P, Tendal B, et al. Effects of glucosamine, chondroitin, or placebo in patients with osteoarthritis of hip or knee: network meta-analysis. BMJ 2010; 341:c4675.

30. Clegg DO, Reda DJ, Harris CL, et al. Glucosamine, chondroitin sulfate, and the two in combination for painful knee osteoarthritis. N Engl J Med 2006;354(8): 795–808.

31. Towheed TE, Maxwell L, Anastassiades TP, et al. Glucosamine therapy for treating osteoarthritis. Cochrane Database Syst Rev 2005;(2):CD002946.

32. Hochberg MC, Martel-Pelletier J, Monfort J, et al. Combined chondroitin sulfate and glucosamine for painful knee osteoarthritis: a multicentre, randomised, double-blind, non-inferiority trial versus celecoxib. Ann Rheum Dis 2016;75(1): 37–44.

33. Rovati LC, Girolami F, D'Amato M, et al. Effects of glucosamine sulfate on the use of rescue non-steroidal anti-inflammatory drugs in knee osteoarthritis: results from the Pharmaco-Epidemiology of GonArthroSis (PEGASus) study. Semin Arthritis Rheum 2016;45(4 Suppl):S34–41.

34. Joshi Jubert N, Rodriguez L, Reverte-Vinaixa MM, et al. Platelet-rich plasma injections for advanced knee osteoarthritis: a prospective, randomized, double-blinded clinical trial. Orthop J Sports Med 2017;5(2). 2325967116689386.

35. Dai WL, Zhou AG, Zhang H, et al. Efficacy of platelet-rich plasma in the treatment of knee osteoarthritis: a meta-analysis of randomized controlled trials. Arthroscopy 2017;33(3):659–70.e1.

36. Campbell KA, Saltzman BM, Mascarenhas R, et al. Does intra-articular platelet-rich plasma injection provide clinically superior outcomes compared with other therapies in the treatment of knee osteoarthritis? A systematic review of overlapping meta-analyses. Arthroscopy 2015;31(11):2213–21.

37. Lui M, Jones CA, Westby MD. Effect of non-surgical, non-pharmacological weight loss interventions in patients who are obese prior to hip and knee arthroplasty surgery: a rapid review. Syst Rev 2015;4:121.

38. Jay R, Lieberman RKA. Perioperative assessment and management. In: Michael AM, Tanzer M, editors. Orthopaedic knowledge update: hip and knee reconstruction 5. Rosemont (IL): American Academy of Orthopaedic Surgeons; 2017. p. 15–26.

39. Verlicchi F, Desalvo F, Zanotti G, et al. Red cell transfusion in orthopaedic surgery: a benchmark study performed combining data from different data sources. Blood Transfus 2011;9(4):383–7.

40. Harris AH, Bowe TR, Gupta S, et al. Hemoglobin A1C as a marker for surgical risk in diabetic patients undergoing total joint arthroplasty. J Arthroplasty 2013;28(8 Suppl):25–9.

41. Giori NJ, Ellerbe LS, Bowe T, et al. Many diabetic total joint arthroplasty candidates are unable to achieve a preoperative hemoglobin A1c goal of 7% or less. J Bone Joint Surg Am 2014;96(6):500–4.

42. Hwang JS, Kim SJ, Bamne AB, et al. Do glycemic markers predict occurrence of complications after total knee arthroplasty in patients with diabetes? Clin Orthop Relat Res 2015;473(5):1726–31.

43. Meding JB, Reddleman K, Keating ME, et al. Total knee replacement in patients with diabetes mellitus. Clin Orthop Relat Res 2003;(416):208–16.

44. Ward DT, Metz LN, Horst PK, et al. Complications of morbid obesity in total joint arthroplasty: risk stratification based on BMI. J Arthroplasty 2015;30(9 Suppl): 42–6.

45. Ogden CL, Carroll MD, Kit BK, et al. Prevalence of childhood and adult obesity in the United States, 2011-2012. JAMA 2014;311(8):806–14.

46. Welton KL, Gagnier JJ, Urquhart AG. Proportion of obese patients presenting to orthopedic total joint arthroplasty clinics. Orthopedics 2016;39(1):e127–33.

47. Workgroup of the American Association of Hip and Knee Surgeons Evidence Based Committee. Obesity and total joint arthroplasty: a literature based review. J Arthroplasty 2013;28(5):714–21.

48. Paxton EW, Inacio MC, Khatod M, et al. Risk calculators predict failures of knee and hip arthroplasties: findings from a large health maintenance organization. Clin Orthop Relat Res 2015;473(12):3965–73.

49. Watts CD, Houdek MT, Wagner ER, et al. Subcutaneous fat thickness is associated with early reoperation and infection after total knee arthroplasty in morbidly obese patients. J Arthroplasty 2016;31(8):1788–91.

50. Sprowls GR, Pruszynski JE, Allen BC. Distribution of subcutaneous fat around the hip in relation to surgical approach for total hip arthroplasty. J Arthroplasty 2016;31(6):1213–7.

51. Jacob AK, Hurley SP, Loughran SM, et al. Continuing clopidogrel during elective total hip and knee arthroplasty: assessment of bleeding risk and adverse outcomes. J Arthroplasty 2014;29(2):325–8.

52. Falck-Ytter Y, Francis CW, Johanson NA, et al. Prevention of VTE in orthopedic surgery patients: antithrombotic therapy and prevention of thrombosis, 9th ed: American College of Chest Physicians Evidence-Based Clinical Practice Guidelines. Chest 2012;141(2 Suppl):e278S–325.

53. American Academy of Orthopaedic Surgeons. Clinical practice guidelines on preventing venous thromboembolic disease in patients undergoing elective hip and knee arthroplasty In: AAOS current guidelines. 2011. Available at: http://www.aaos.org/research/guidelines/VTE/VTE_full_guideline.pdf. Accessed March 23, 2017.

54. Sehat KR, Evans RL, Newman JH. Hidden blood loss following hip and knee arthroplasty. Correct management of blood loss should take hidden loss into account. J Bone Joint Surg Br 2004;86(4):561–5.

55. Viola J, Gomez MM, Restrepo C, et al. Preoperative anemia increases postoperative complications and mortality following total joint arthroplasty. J Arthroplasty 2015;30(5):846–8.

56. Spahn DR. Anemia and patient blood management in hip and knee surgery: a systematic review of the literature. Anesthesiology 2010;113(2):482–95.

57. Yatin Kirane FDC. Blood management. In: Michael AM, Tanzer M, editors. Orthopaedic knowledge update: hip and knee reconstruction 5. Rosemont (IL): American Academy of Orthopaedic Surgeons; 2017. p. 27–44.

58. Holt JB, Miller BJ, Callaghan JJ, et al. Minimizing blood transfusion in total hip and knee arthroplasty through a multimodal approach. J Arthroplasty 2016; 31(2):378–82.

59. Serrano Mateo L, Goudarz Mehdikhani K, Caceres L, et al. Topical tranexamic acid may improve early functional outcomes of primary total knee arthroplasty. J Arthroplasty 2016;31(7):1449–52.

60. Tengborn L, Blomback M, Berntorp E. Tranexamic acid–an old drug still going strong and making a revival. Thromb Res 2015;135(2):231–42.

61. Giles R, Scuderi HDC, Dodd CA. Minimally invasive surgical approaches to the knee arthroplasty. In: Michael AM, Tanzer M, editors. Orthopaedic knowledge update: hip and knee reconstruction 5. Rosemont (IL): American Academy of Orthopaedic Surgeons; 2017. p. 95–103.

62. Haas SB, Cook S, Beksac B. Minimally invasive total knee replacement through a mini midvastus approach: a comparative study. Clin Orthop Relat Res 2004;(428):68–73.

63. Chen AF, Alan RK, Redziniak DE, et al. Quadriceps sparing total knee replacement. The initial experience with results at two to four years. J Bone Joint Surg Br 2006;88(11):1448–53.

64. Dutton AQ, Yeo SJ, Yang KY, et al. Computer-assisted minimally invasive total knee arthroplasty compared with standard total knee arthroplasty. A prospective, randomized study. J Bone Joint Surg Am 2008;90(1):2–9.

65. McAllister CM, Stepanian JD. The impact of minimally invasive surgical techniques on early range of motion after primary total knee arthroplasty. J Arthroplasty 2008;23(1):10–8.

66. Dutton AQ, Yeo SJ. Computer-assisted minimally invasive total knee arthroplasty compared with standard total knee arthroplasty. Surgical technique. J Bone Joint Surg Am 2009;91(Suppl 2 Pt 1):116–30.

67. Bonutti PM, Zywiel MG, Ulrich SD, et al. A comparison of subvastus and midvastus approaches in minimally invasive total knee arthroplasty. J Bone Joint Surg Am 2010;92(3):575–82.

68. Nestor BJ, Toulson CE, Backus SI, et al. Mini-midvastus vs standard medial parapatellar approach: a prospective, randomized, double-blinded study in patients undergoing bilateral total knee arthroplasty. J Arthroplasty 2010;25(6 Suppl):5–11, 11.e1.

69. Bourke MG, Sclavos EK, Jull GA, et al. A comparison of patellar vascularity between the medial parapatellar and subvastus approaches in total knee arthroplasty. J Arthroplasty 2012;27(6):1123–7.e1.

70. Heekin RD, Fokin AA. Mini-midvastus versus mini-medial parapatellar approach for minimally invasive total knee arthroplasty: outcomes pendulum is at equilibrium. J Arthroplasty 2014;29(2):339–42.

71. Liu TK, Chen SH. Simultaneous bilateral total knee arthroplasty in a single procedure. Int Orthop 1998;22(6):390–3.

72. Leonard L, Williamson DM, Ivory JP, et al. An evaluation of the safety and efficacy of simultaneous bilateral total knee arthroplasty. J Arthroplasty 2003; 18(8):972–8.

73. Fu D, Li G, Chen K, et al. Comparison of clinical outcome between simultaneous-bilateral and staged-bilateral total knee arthroplasty: a systematic review of retrospective studies. J Arthroplasty 2013;28(7):1141–7.

74. Odum SM, Troyer JL, Kelly MP, et al. A cost-utility analysis comparing the cost-effectiveness of simultaneous and staged bilateral total knee arthroplasty. J Bone Joint Surg Am 2013;95(16):1441–9.

75. Restrepo C, Parvizi J, Dietrich T, et al. Safety of simultaneous bilateral total knee arthroplasty. A meta-analysis. J Bone Joint Surg Am 2007;89(6):1220–6.

76. Browne JA, Pagnano MW. Surgical technique: a simple soft-tissue-only repair of the capsule and external rotators in posterior-approach THA. Clin Orthop Relat Res 2012;470(2):511–5.

77. Zhang D, Chen L, Peng K, et al. Effectiveness and safety of the posterior approach with soft tissue repair for primary total hip arthroplasty: a meta-analysis. Orthop Traumatol Surg Res 2015;101(1):39–44.

78. Berstock JR, Blom AW, Beswick AD. A systematic review and meta-analysis of complications following the posterior and lateral surgical approaches to total hip arthroplasty. Ann R Coll Surg Engl 2015;97(1):11–6.

79. Hozack W, Duncan CP, Herman A, et al. Surgical approaches and bearing surfaces. In: Michael AM, Tanzer M, editors. Orthopaedic knowledge update: hip and knee reconstruction 5. Rosemont (IL): American Academy of Orthopaedic Surgeons; 2017. p. 345–66.

80. Restrepo C, Parvizi J, Pour AE, et al. Prospective randomized study of two surgical approaches for total hip arthroplasty. J Arthroplasty 2010;25(5):671–9.e1.

81. Higgins BT, Barlow DR, Heagerty NE, et al. Anterior vs. posterior approach for total hip arthroplasty, a systematic review and meta-analysis. J Arthroplasty 2015;30(3):419–34.

82. Yue C, Kang P, Pei F. Comparison of direct anterior and lateral approaches in total hip arthroplasty: a systematic review and meta-analysis (PRISMA). Medicine 2015;94(50):e2126.

83. Viktor E, Krebs AM, Slif D, et al. Complications of knee arthroplasty. In: Michael AM, Tanzer M, editors. Orthopaedic knowledge update: hip and knee reconstruction 5. Rosemont (IL): American Academy of Orthopaedic Surgeons; 2017. p. 233–66.

84. Albers A, Kheir M, Daivajna S, et al. Complications of total hip arthroplasty. In: Michael AM, Tanzer M, editors. Orthopaedic knowledge update: hip and knee

reconstruction 5. Rosemont (IL): American Academy of Orthopaedic Surgeons; 2017. p. 473–506.

85. Johnston AT, Tsiridis E, Eyres KS, et al. Periprosthetic fractures in the distal femur following total knee replacement: a review and guide to management. Knee 2012;19(3):156–62.

86. Ponzio DY, Shahi A, Park AG, et al. Intraoperative proximal femoral fracture in primary cementless total hip arthroplasty. J Arthroplasty 2015;30(8):1418–22.

87. Haidukewych GJ, Jacofsky DJ, Hanssen AD, et al. Intraoperative fractures of the acetabulum during primary total hip arthroplasty. J Bone Joint Surg Am 2006;88(9):1952–6.

88. Kurtz SM, Lau E, Watson H, et al. Economic burden of periprosthetic joint infection in the United States. J Arthroplasty 2012;27(8 Suppl):61–5.e1.

89. Kamath AF, Ong KL, Lau E, et al. Quantifying the burden of revision total joint arthroplasty for periprosthetic infection. J Arthroplasty 2015;30(9):1492–7.

90. Hackett DJ, Rothenberg AC, Chen AF, et al. The economic significance of orthopaedic infections. J Am Acad Orthop Surg 2015;23(Suppl):S1–7.

91. Khan M, Osman K, Green G, et al. The epidemiology of failure in total knee arthroplasty: avoiding your next revision. Bone Joint J 2016;98-b(1 Suppl A): 105–12.

92. Thiele K, Perka C, Matziolis G, et al. Current failure mechanisms after knee arthroplasty have changed: polyethylene wear is less common in revision surgery. J Bone Joint Surg Am 2015;97(9):715–20.

93. Sharkey PF, Lichstein PM, Shen C, et al. Why are total knee arthroplasties failing today–has anything changed after 10 years? J Arthroplasty 2014;29(9):1774–8.

94. Schroer WC, Berend KR, Lombardi AV, et al. Why are total knees failing today? Etiology of total knee revision in 2010 and 2011. J Arthroplasty 2013;28(8 Suppl):116–9.

95. Malkani AL, Ong KL, Lau E, et al. Early- and late-term dislocation risk after primary hip arthroplasty in the Medicare population. J Arthroplasty 2010;25(6 Suppl):21–5.

96. Sculco PK, Pagnano MW. Perioperative solutions for rapid recovery joint arthroplasty: get ahead and stay ahead. J Arthroplasty 2015;30(4):518–20.

97. Filardo G, Roffi A, Merli G, et al. Patient kinesiophobia affects both recovery time and final outcome after total knee arthroplasty. Knee Surg Sports Traumatol Arthrosc 2016;24(10):3322–8.

98. Lombardi AV. Outpatient total knee arthroplasty. In: Michael AM, Tanzer M, editors. Orthopaedic knowledge update: hip and knee reconstruction 5. Rosemont (IL): American Academy of Orthopaedic Surgeons; 2017. p. 223–32.

99. Helwani MA, Avidan MS, Ben Abdallah A, et al. Effects of regional versus general anesthesia on outcomes after total hip arthroplasty: a retrospective propensity-matched cohort study. J Bone Joint Surg Am 2015;97(3):186–93.

100. Pugely AJ, Martin CT, Gao Y, et al. Differences in short-term complications between spinal and general anesthesia for primary total knee arthroplasty. J Bone Joint Surg Am 2013;95(3):193–9.

101. Spangehl MJ, Clarke HD, Hentz JG, et al. The Chitranjan Ranawat Award: periarticular injections and femoral & sciatic blocks provide similar pain relief after TKA: a randomized clinical trial. Clin Orthop Relat Res 2015;473(1):45–53.

102. Ng FY, Ng JK, Chiu KY, et al. Multimodal periarticular injection vs continuous femoral nerve block after total knee arthroplasty: a prospective, crossover, randomized clinical trial. J Arthroplasty 2012;27(6):1234–8.

103. Chan EY, Fransen M, Sathappan S, et al. Comparing the analgesia effects of single-injection and continuous femoral nerve blocks with patient controlled analgesia after total knee arthroplasty. J Arthroplasty 2013;28(4):608–13.
104. Buhagiar MA, Naylor JM, Harris IA, et al. Effect of inpatient rehabilitation vs a monitored home-based program on mobility in patients with total knee arthroplasty: the HIHO Randomized Clinical Trial. JAMA 2017;317(10):1037–46.
105. Mahomed NN, Davis AM, Hawker G, et al. Inpatient compared with home-based rehabilitation following primary unilateral total hip or knee replacement: a randomized controlled trial. J Bone Joint Surg Am 2008;90(8):1673–80.
106. Starks I, Wainwright TW, Lewis J, et al. Older patients have the most to gain from orthopaedic enhanced recovery programmes. Age Ageing 2014;43(5):642–8.
107. Malviya A, Martin K, Harper I, et al. Enhanced recovery program for hip and knee replacement reduces death rate. Acta Orthop 2011;82(5):577–81.
108. Belmar CJ, Barth P, Lonner JH, et al. Total knee arthroplasty in patients 90 years of age and older. J Arthroplasty 1999;14(8):911–4.
109. Berend ME, Thong AE, Faris GW, et al. Total joint arthroplasty in the extremely elderly: hip and knee arthroplasty after entering the 89th year of life. J Arthroplasty 2003;18(7):817–21.
110. Joshi AB, Gill G. Total knee arthroplasty in nonagenarians. J Arthroplasty 2002; 17(6):681–4.
111. Pagnano MW, McLamb LA, Trousdale RT. Total knee arthroplasty for patients 90 years of age and older. Clin Orthop Relat Res 2004;(418):179–83.
112. Brander VA, Malhotra S, Jet J, et al. Outcome of hip and knee arthroplasty in persons aged 80 years and older. Clin Orthop Relat Res 1997;(345):67–78.
113. Huddleston JM, Long KH, Naessens JM, et al. Medical and surgical comanagement after elective hip and knee arthroplasty: a randomized, controlled trial. Ann Intern Med 2004;141(1):28–38.
114. Walke LM, Rosenthal RA, Trentalange M, et al. Restructuring care for older adults undergoing surgery: preliminary data from the Co-Management of Older Operative Patients En Route Across Treatment Environments (CO-OPERATE) model of care. J Am Geriatr Soc 2014;62(11):2185–90.
115. Arnold JB, Walters JL, Ferrar KE. Does physical activity increase after total hip or knee arthroplasty for osteoarthritis? A systematic review. J Orthop Sports Phys Ther 2016;46(6):431–42.
116. Harding P, Holland AE, Delany C, et al. Do activity levels increase after total hip and knee arthroplasty? Clin Orthop Relat Res 2014;472(5):1502–11.
117. Webber SC, Strachan SM, Pachu NS. Sedentary behavior, cadence, and physical activity outcomes after knee arthroplasty. Med Sci Sports Exerc 2017;49(6): 1057–65.
118. Chang MJ, Kang YG, Chung BJ, et al. Why patients do not participate in sports activities after total knee arthroplasty. Orthop J Sports Med 2015;3(4). 2325967115579171.
119. Bloomfield MR, Hozack WJ. Total hip and knee replacement in the mature athlete. Sports Health 2014;6(1):78–80.
120. Meira EP, Zeni J Jr. Sports participation following total hip arthroplasty. Int J Sports Phys Ther 2014;9(6):839–50.
121. Vogel LA, Carotenuto G, Basti JJ, et al. Physical activity after total joint arthroplasty. Sports Health 2011;3(5):441–50.
122. Hernandez VH, Ong A, Orozco F, et al. When is it safe for patients to drive after right total hip arthroplasty? J Arthroplasty 2015;30(4):627–30.

Rehabilitation Needs of the Elderly Patient with Cancer

Jesuel Padro-Guzman, MD[a,b,*], Jennifer P. Moody, MD[c], Jessica L. Au, MD[c,d]

KEYWORDS

• Cancer • Rehabilitation • Geriatric • Function

KEY POINTS

• The challenge for a physiatrist is to anticipate and coordinate treatments for elders suffering from cancer or the effects of its treatments.
• The physician should anticipate changes in clinical status and must adjust rehabilitation goals accordingly.
• Treatment options and rehabilitation goals should be tailored to help maximize quality of life in these patients.

BACKGROUND

As the average age in the United States population grows older, the prevalence of cancer in the elderly is more apparent. It is estimated that, by 2030, 70% of all cancers will be within people older than 65,[1] with prostate, breast, lung, and colorectal cancers being the most common.[2] This estimated increase in cancer prevalence highlights the connection of carcinogenesis with aging.

Elderly patients with cancer are consistently undertreated or alternatively treated when compared with younger patients. For example, patients with breast or stage II colorectal cancers are less likely to receive chemotherapy and radiation as age advances. Radical prostatectomy is considered the gold standard of curative treatment in prostate cancer, yet, as patient age, the rates of prostatectomy decrease accompanied by an increase in rates of radiation and more conservative management.[3] Studies across many types of cancer consistently reach the same conclusion: we often treat

The authors have nothing to disclose.
[a] Department of Neurology, Memorial Sloan Kettering Cancer Center, 1275 York Avenue, New York, NY 10065, USA; [b] Division of Rehabilitation Medicine, Weill Cornell Medicine, 525 East 68th Street, New York, NY 10065, USA; [c] Department of Rehabilitation Medicine, New York Presbyterian Hospital, Harkness Pavilion, 180 Fort Washington Avenue, New York, NY 10032, USA; [d] Hudson Spine & Pain Medicine, 281 Broadway, New York, NY 10007, USA
* Corresponding author. Department of Neurology, Memorial Sloan Kettering Cancer Center, and 1275 York Avenue, New York, NY 10065
E-mail address: padroguj@mskcc.org

Phys Med Rehabil Clin N Am 28 (2017) 811–819
http://dx.doi.org/10.1016/j.pmr.2017.06.012
1047-9651/17/© 2017 Elsevier Inc. All rights reserved.
pmr.theclinics.com

geriatric patients differently than our younger populations. The reason for this disparity is multifactorial, but is largely a fear of intolerance to more aggressive therapies in the elderly. Geriatric patients are physiologically more susceptible to complications owing to decreased cardiac reserve, decreased intestinal motility, decreased lung vital capacity with impaired gas exchange, diminished glomerular filtration rate leading to increased drug half-life, changes in arterial pressure and cerebral blood flow, and disequilibrium resulting in confusion, syncope, and falls. The challenge for a physiatrist is to anticipate and coordinate treatments for elders suffering from cancer or the effects of its treatments. In the majority of these cases, the physician observes an amplification of symptoms and abrupt change in functional status with slower return to baseline.

PHYSIATRIC ASSESSMENT OF THE ELDERLY PATIENTS WITH CANCER

Pretreatment performance level assessment should include level of independence, need for mobility aids and adaptive equipment, and history of falls. The physiatrist should investigate, in great detail, the types of cancer treatment undergone: surgery, radiation, chemotherapy, and immunotherapy, as well as maintenance therapy. Enquiring about social support, recreational activities, emotional needs, and cognition is highly important because these factors will affect the rehabilitation program directly. In addition to history and comprehensive physical examination, it is useful to include standardized functional status measurements. Examples include the Timed Get-Up and-Go and the unipedal stance test, which help to identify patients at risk for falls.[4,5] Addressing fall risk is an important task for the rehabilitation team. Elderly patients with cancer may have a higher risk for falls compared with elderly patients without cancer.[6] Reducing or preventing falls will improve morbidity and mortality in this patient group.

The Comprehensive Geriatric Assessment (CGA) is an assessment tool that gives physicians and other caregivers a comprehensive analysis of the overall global health of a geriatric patient. This assessment includes all aspects of health, including functionality, comorbid medical conditions, nutrition, cognition, psychological status, polypharmacy, social support, financial status, and geriatric conditions. This assessment divides patients into 3 broad categories: Fit, Vulnerable, and Frail.

Fit patients include:

- Patients in good to excellent health,
- Patients who are functionally independent,
- Patients with no medical comorbidities, and
- Patients with no geriatric conditions.

Vulnerable patients include:

- Patients in fair to good health,
- Patients who are independent in their activities of daily living (ADLs), but may need assistance in some instrumental ADLs,
- Patients with fewer than 3 mild comorbidities, and
- Patients with mild geriatric conditions including mild depression, mild cognitive deficits, or risk for malnutrition.

Frail patients include:

- Patients with overall poor health,
- Patients who require assistance in some or all ADLs,
- Patients with 3 or more medical comorbidities or 1 life-threatening comorbidity, and
- Patients with geriatric conditions.

Studies have shown that CGA is a strong predictor of mortality in patients with cancer, with fit patients having significantly higher survival rates than frail patients.[7,8] A higher degree of frailty predicts a higher risk for mortality, regardless of patient age or disease stage. Additionally, the CGA has been shown to be a useful tool in helping to determine which patients are more likely to be able to tolerate and benefit from more aggressive treatments.[9] The evidence that exists shows clear differences between frail and fit patients in mortality and their ability to tolerate aggressive treatment; however, where vulnerable patients fit in is less clear. However, considering the evidence that rehabilitation has been shown to improve functional status,[10,11] it is reasonable to hypothesize that many of the patients in the vulnerable functionality category may benefit from rehabilitation to increase functionality and allow them to move from the vulnerable to the fit category, thereby availing them to more treatment options. A proposed use of the CGA in cancer treatment approach can be seen in **Fig. 1**. This suggested treatment algorithm from Kilari and Mohile suggests using rehabilitation to attempt increase patients' functionality and allow them to move from being vulnerable to fit, in hopes of increasing their chances of survival and treatment tolerance.

By using the CGA in geriatric patients, we can better understand a patient's global health needs, and can more accurately determine which patients are likely to benefit from rehabilitation before cancer treatment.

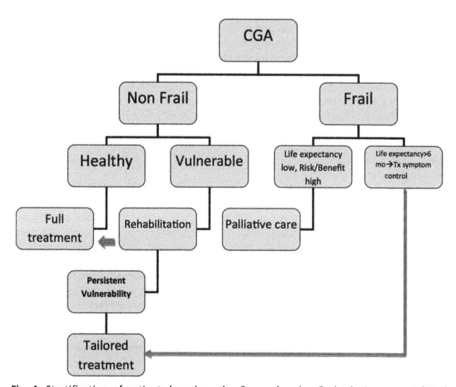

Fig. 1. Stratification of patients based on the Comprehensive Geriatric Assessment (CGA) and suggested treatment algorithm. (*From* Kilari D, Mohile S. Management of cancer in the older adult. Clin Geriatr Med 2012;28(1):33–49; with permission.)

PAIN IN THE GERIATRIC PATIENT WITH CANCER

Pain is a common complaint among patients with cancer, and is even more common in the geriatric population.[12] Up to two-thirds of patients with cancer experience pain occurring from cancer or as a result of its treatment. Geriatric patients with cancer are also likely to have pain from sources other than cancer, including degenerative changes of the joints and spine.[13] When treating pain in the geriatric population, it is important to be conscious of polypharmacy and altered medication metabolism.

Geriatric patients with cancer, like all other patients, can experience both nociceptive and neuropathic pain. When managing nociceptive pain, acetaminophen is considered the preferred medication for mild to moderate pain, because it is generally considered safe in elderly patients when doses do not exceed 3000 to 4000 mg. When using acetaminophen, patients should be educated on liver toxicity and need to be made aware that many over-the-counter pain medications contain acetaminophen. Nonsteroidal antiinflammatory drugs (NSAIDs) are another alternative to opioids, and have been shown to be particularly beneficial for patients with bone pain. However, NSAIDs have been linked to gastrointestinal bleeds, renal toxicity, myocardial infarction, and stroke in elderly patients and should be avoided in patients with congestive heart failure, peptic ulcer disease, bleeding tendency, or renal insufficiency.[13,14] When prescribing NSAIDs, practitioners should also prescribe medications such as proton pump inhibitors or H2 blockers to aid in protection of the gastrointestinal tract. Opioids should be used with caution in geriatric patients, because elderly patients are more prone to neuropsychiatric sensitivity (including delirium, sedation, hallucinations, and confusion), respiratory depression, urinary retention, and constipation associated with opioid usage.[12] However, opioids are generally well-tolerated in elderly patients when titrated properly. When titrating opioid medications, it is important to keep in mind that half-life of medications may be longer than in younger patients, so titrating slowly is preferred. Patients generally develop a tolerance to drowsiness and confusion after a few days of use. However, patients do not develop tolerance to constipation and an aggressive bowel regimen should always be used in conjunction with opioids, particularly in elderly patients.[11] The author's preference is to avoid opioids as much as possible. If opioids are prescribed, a plan to taper down should be establish with promptitude. Topical analgesics such as lidocaine patches or creams are another safe option for treatment of both nociceptive and neuropathic pain.

A large number of patients with cancer treated with certain types of chemotherapy develop peripheral neuropathy and significant neuropathic pain. In treatment of neuropathic pain, medications such as anti-epileptics (gabapentin, pregabalin) and antidepressants (tricyclic antidepressants, selective norepinephrine inhibitors) are effective. These medications must be used in caution in the geriatric patient, because tricyclic antidepressants have significant anticholinergic side effects resulting in cognitive changes and are generally contraindicated in elderly patients. Antiepileptic medications such as gabapentin and pregabalin are better tolerated, but should be renally dosed and slowly titrated in elderly patients.[13] selective norepinephrine inhibitors are generally well-tolerated in older patients and are also effective in treating neuropathic pain.

Treatments such as physical therapy, psychotherapy, massage, herbal supplements, injections, or acupuncture should be considered as an alternative or in conjunction with medications in geriatric patients. Physical therapy and exercise have been shown to improve pain and fatigue in patients with cancer.[15] A large number of patients with breast cancer who have undergone mastectomy will develop shoulder dysfunction and chest wall pain. Image-guided injection, antiinflammatory medications, and a supervised rehabilitation program that includes stretching of pectoralis, muscle strengthening, soft tissue mobilization, and postural and biomechanics training are highly effective in treating these issues.[16,17]

Massage has been shown to be effective in improving quality of life in patients with end-stage cancer, and improves functionality in patients with neck pain.[18] There have been some early studies and case reports suggesting that acupuncture may be a beneficial adjunctive treatment for chemotherapy-induced peripheral neuropathy in patients with multiple myeloma[19] and in acute and postoperative pain. The idea of acupuncture to manage painful disorders in the elderly is appealing, because it might reduce polypharmacy and potential side effects of pain control medications. Herbal supplements such as curcumin and ginger are being used more commonly in treatment of pain, and are often used in patients unable to tolerate NSAIDs, because there is evidence to suggest that these supplements have similar efficacy to antiinflammatory and analgesic agents.[20] However, the physiatrist needs to make sure there no interactions with these supplements and other medications or chemotherapies.

FATIGUE

Cancer-related fatigue (CRF) is one of the most common and debilitating symptoms experienced by oncology patients, occurring in 70% to 100% of patients.[21] It is defined by the National Comprehensive Cancer Network as a "distressing persistent, subjective sense of tiredness or exhaustion related to cancer or cancer treatment that is not proportional to recent activity and interferes with usual functioning."[22] Unlike healthy individuals, this fatigue does not improve with rest. Several biologic mechanisms for causing fatigue have been proposed, including serotonin dysregulation, endocrine dysfunction, circadian rhythm disruption, and cytokine dysregulation, but the actual mechanism remains unknown. In the elderly patient, fatigue can lead to functional decline, which leads to increased morbidity and mortality, and has further psychological, social, and economic impacts. Any potential reversible causes for fatigue should first be addressed when assessing fatigue in oncology patients. This is particular important in the elderly patient with cancer, because CRF can severely affect concentration, memory, and mood and consequently reduce cognitive performance.

Both nonpharmacologic and medications can be used in treatment of CRF. Nonpharmacologic treatments include strengthening and endurance-based exercise programs, psychosocial interventions (including fatigue education, stress management, relaxation techniques, and support groups), and complementary therapies including acupuncture, acupressure, yoga, and massage therapy. Many studies have been performed examining the benefits of exercise on fatigue, and the general consensus seems to be that exercise is safe and effective at reducing fatigue and improving quality of life in patients with cancer, as well as in preventing further decline in functional performance.[22,23]

Pharmacologic treatments used for CRF include psychostimulants, such as methylphenidate and modafinil, and antidepressants including paroxetine and bupropion. Paroxetine has been shown to be effective in patients with fatigue, primarily when fatigue is secondary to depression. Bupropion is thought to have psychostimulant effects, which aid with fatigue.[24] Some studies have suggested that ginseng used at 1000 to 2000 mg/d may improve treatment-related fatigue in patients with cancer.[25]

LYMPHEDEMA

A large number of patients with cancer who have undergone surgical resection of lymph nodes will develop lymphedema. Risk factors for the development of lymphedema include extent and location of the surgical intervention, radiation location, infection, weight gain, and age.[26] Lymphedema frequently causes heaviness of the affected limb, leading to severe morbidity and impairment of ADLs. Overall, about 30% of patients with breast cancer will develop breast cancer–related lymphedema. The incidence and severity increases with age, making elderly patients more prone to developing this condition.[12] In geriatric patients who are already at risk for developing functional impairments, early and effective prevention and treatment for lymphedema is essential. Exercise has been shown to enhance lymph flow and improve protein resorption, making it an essential part of any treatment program.[26,27] Getting these patients into lymphedema therapy early on to guide in exercise, provide low-stretch wrapping of the affected limb, and teach manual lymphedema drainage massage, as well as fitting and obtaining appropriately fitting compression garments is extremely important in the elderly population. Additionally, it is important to educate patients and caregivers on proper skin care for the affected limb, including washing with soap and water and applying an alcohol free-moisturizer to prevent cellulitis and lymphangitis.

Conservative management of lymphedema has been the gold standard of lymphedema treatment for many years. In recent years, microsurgical approaches to treating lymphedema such as vascularized lymph node transfers, lymphaticovenous anastomoses, lymphatic–venous–lymphatic plasties, and lymphaticolymphatic grafts are starting to be used and have shown to be efficacious in patients with severe lymphedema.[28] However, studies performed thus far have been small studies and generally have not represented the elderly population. It is unclear at this time whether there is a role for the surgical treatment of lymphedema in the geriatric patient, but it is an option to consider in a fit elderly patient with severe lymphedema who may be an appropriate surgical candidate.

BONE HEALTH

Bone health is of significant concern in the geriatric patient with cancer. Elderly patients are at increased risk of developing osteoporosis and osteopenia, which carries a high risk of morbidity and mortality. Many of the treatments used to treat breast cancer, including aromatase inhibitors, doxorubicin, methotrexate, and glucocorticoids, can cause or worsen osteoporosis. Aromatase inhibitors and chemotherapy-induced ovarian failure can lead to rapid bone loss. Similarly, patients with prostate cancer are also at high risk of developing osteoporosis owing to iatrogenic induction of a hypogonadal state in patients undergoing androgen deprivation therapy.[29,30] Other causes leading to bone loss in patients with cancer include bone marrow transplantation, chronic corticosteroid treatment, supraphysiologic thyroid hormone suppression therapy, and chemotherapy-induced bone cell toxicity. Like any other patient, elderly patients with cancer should always undergo workup for secondary causes of bone loss.

Women with newly diagnosed breast cancer are at significant risk for vertebral fractures, and have been shown to be 5 times more likely to develop a vertebral fracture than the general population. Women with breast cancer recurrence are 20 times more likely than the general population to develop vertebral fracture.[30] Thus, when evaluating a patient with breast cancer and back pain, particularly in the elderly, a vertebral fracture should always be high on the differential diagnosis.

Treatment recommendations include an exercise program of at least 30 minutes of weight bearing activity daily, as well as calcium and vitamin D supplementation owing to evidence to support bone mineral density preservation and reduced risk of fracture in patients with osteoporosis. Trials using bisphosphonates in patients with breast cancer have demonstrated benefits of prophylactic bisphosphonate use in preventing osteoporosis.[31] Bisphosphonates have similarly shown benefits in increasing femoral and lumbar spine bone mineral density and decreasing risk of osteoporosis in patients with prostate cancer on androgen deprivation therapy.[29] However, bisphosphonates do carry risks, including fatigue, bone pain, and anemia, which can be increased in the elderly owing to decreased renal clearance. Denosumab is another treatment option that has shown efficacy in increasing bone mineral density and decreasing vertebral fracture rates in patients with prostate cancer on androgen deprivation therapy. Denosumab does carry a risk of causing hypocalcemia, and may cause nonspecific symptoms in elderly patients.[32–35]

SUMMARY

Physiatrist taking care of the geriatric patient with cancer should be able to manage an array of conditions that might present from diagnosis throughout completion of treatments and beyond. The elderly cancer population is at greater risk of functional impairments. The physician should anticipate changes in clinical status and must adjust rehabilitation goals accordingly. Treatment options and rehabilitation goals should be tailored to help maximize quality of life in these patients.

REFERENCES

1. Smith BD, Smith GL, Hurria A, et al. Future of cancer incidence in the United States: burdens upon an aging, changing nation. J Clin Oncol 2009;27:2758–65.
2. Siegel RL, Miller KD, Jemal A. Cancer statistic, 2016. CA Cancer J Clin 2016; 66(1):7–30, 2015 American Cancer Society.
3. Chen RC, Royce TJ, Extermann M, et al. Impact of age and comorbidity on treatment and outcomes in elderly cancer patients. Semin Radiat Oncol 2012;22(4): 265–71.
4. Hurvitz EA, Richardson JK, Werner RA, et al. Unipedal stance testing as an indicator of fall risk among older outpatients. Arch Phys Med Rehabil 2000;81(5): 587–91.
5. Podsiadlo D, Richardson S. The timed "Up & Go": a test of basic functional mobility for frail elderly persons. J Am Geriatr Soc 1991;39(2):142–8.
6. Bylow K, Dale W, Mustian K, et al. Falls and physical performance deficits in older patients with prostate cancer undergoing androgen deprivation therapy. Urology 2008;72(2):422–7.
7. Liu J, Extermann M. Comprehensive Geriatric Assessment and its clinical impact in oncology. Clin Geriatr Med 2012;28(1):19–31.
8. Arnoldi E, Dieli M, Mangia M, et al. Comprehensive Geriatric Assessment in elderly cancer patients: an experience in an outpatient population. Tumori 2007;93:23–5.
9. Stotter A, Reed MW, Gray LJ, et al. Comprehensive Geriatric Assessment and predicted 3-year survival in treatment planning for frail patients with early breast cancer. Br J Surg 2015;102(5):525–33.
10. Marciniak CM, Sliwa JA, Spill G, et al. Functional outcome following rehabilitation of the cancer patient. Arch Phys Med Rehabil 1996;77(1):54–7.
11. Tay SS, Lim PA, Ng YS. Poster 21: functional outcomes of cancer patients in an inpatient rehabilitation setting. Arch Phys Med Rehabil 2007;88(9):E15–6.
12. Gosain R, Pollock Y, Jain D. Age-related disparity: breast cancer in the elderly. Curr Oncol Rep 2016;18:69.

13. Alexander K, Goldberg J, Korc-Grodzicki B. Palliative care and symptom management in older patients with cancer. Clin Geriatr Med 2016;32(1):45–62.
14. Lee TY, Ganz SB. Geriatric issues in cancer rehabilitation. In: Stubblefield MD, O'Dell MW, editors. Cancer rehabilitation: principles and practice, vol. 69. New York: Demos Medical Publishing; 2009. p. 869–80.
15. Gracey JH, Watson M, Payne C. Translation research: 'back on track', a multiprofessional rehabilitation service for cancer-related fatigue. BMJ Support Palliat Care 2016;6(1):94–6.
16. Okur SC, Ozyemisci-Taskiran O, Pekindogan Y, et al. Ultrasound-guided block of the suprascapular nerve in breast cancer survivors with limited shoulder motion-case series. Pain Physician 2017;20:E233–9.
17. Padro-Guzman J. Managing upper extremity dysfunction in breast cancer survivors. American Society of Clinical Oncology Post. Available at: http://www.ascopost.com/issues/july-10-2016/managing-upper-extremity-dysfunction-in-breast-cancer-survivors. Accessed July 10, 2016.
18. Lopez-Sendin N, Alburquerque-Sendin F, Cleland JA, et al. Effects of physical therapy on pain and mood in patients with terminal cancer: a pilot randomized clinical trial. J Altern Complement Med 2012;18(5):480–6.
19. Garcia MK, Cohen L, Guo Y, et al. Electroacupuncture for thalidomide/bortezomib-induced peripheral neuropathy in multiple myeloma: a feasibility study. J Hematol Oncol 2014;7:41.
20. Leong M, Smith TJ, Rowland-Seymour A. Complementary and integrative medicine for older adults in palliative care. Clin Geriatr Med 2015;31(2):177–91.
21. Franklin DJ, Packel L. Cancer-related fatigue. In: Stubblefield MD, O'Dell MW, editors. Cancer rehabilitation: principles and practice, vol. 73. New York: Demos Medical Publishing; 2009. p. 929–40.
22. Clinical Practice Guidelines in Oncology: Cancer-related fatigue. National Comprehensive Cancer Network. 2011. Available at: http://www.nccn.org/professionals/physician_gls/f_guidelines.asp. Accessed May 23, 2013.
23. Groeneveldt L, Mein G, Garrod R, et al. A Mixed exercise training programme is feasible and safe and may improve quality of life and muscle strength in multiple myeloma survivors. BMC Cancer 2013;13:31.
24. Marrow GR. Differential effects of paroxetine on fatigue and depression: double randomized trial. J Clin Oncol 2013;21:4635–41.
25. Barton DL, Soori GS, Bauer BA, et al. Pilot study of Panax quinquefolius (American ginseng) to improve cancer-related fatigue: a randomized, double-blind, dose-finding evaluation: NCCTG trial N03CA. Support Care Cancer 2010;18(2):179–87.
26. Strick DM, Gamble GL. Lymphedema in the cancer patient. In: Stubblefield MD, O'Dell MW, editors. Cancer rehabilitation: principles and practice, vol. 79. New York: Demos Medical Publishing; 2009. p. 1011–22.
27. Balci LF, et al. Breast cancer-related lymphedema in elderly patients. Geriatr Rehabil 2012;28(4):243–53.
28. Dionyssiou D, Demiri E, Tsimponis A, et al. A randomized control study of treating secondary stage II breast cancer-related lymphedema with free lymph node transfer. Breast Cancer Res Treat 2016;156(1):73–9.
29. Tay KJ, Moul JW, Armstrong AJ. Management of prostate cancer in the elderly. Clin Geriatr Med 2016;32(1):113–32.
30. Farooki A, Rimner HC. Osteoporosis in cancer. In: Stubblefield MD, O'Dell MW, editors. Cancer rehabilitation: principles and practice, vol. 59. New York: Demos Medical Publishing; 2009. p. 753–71.

31. Majithia N, Atherton PJ, Lafky JM. Zoledronic acid for treatment of osteopenia and osteoporosis in women with primary breast cancer undergoing adjuvant aromatase inhibitor therapy: a 5-year follow-up. Support Care Cancer 2016;24(3): 1219–26.

32. Serpa Neto A, Tobias-Machado M, Esteves MAP, et al. Bisphosphonate therapy in patients under androgen deprivation therapy for prostate cancer: a systematic review and meta-analysis. Prostate Cancer Prostatic Dis 2012;15(1):36–44.

33. Hoffe S, Balducci L. Cancer and age: general considerations. Clin Geriatr Med 2012;28(1):1–18.

34. Li D, de Glas NA, Hurria A. Cancer and aging: general principles, biology, and geriatric assessment. Clin Geriatr Med 2016;32(1):1–15.

35. Korc-Grodzicki B, Wallace JA, Rodin MB, et al. Cancer in long-term care. Clin Geriatr Med 2011;27(2):301–27.

Aging with Spinal Cord Injury: An Update

Joel E. Frontera, MD*, Patrick Mollett, DO

KEYWORDS

- Spinal cord injury • Life expectancy • Quality of life • Disability • Complications

KEY POINTS

- Persons with spinal cord injury (SCI) are living longer compared with 50 years ago. The average age of injury is trending toward older individuals.
- There is a significant variation in mortality among persons with SCI.
- Healthy SCI individuals tend to have better quality of life (QoL) measures than expected.
- Secondary health issues after SCI are affecting patient's QoL and social participation.
- All organ systems are in some way affected after SCI.

INTRODUCTION

According to the National Spinal Cord Injury Statistical Center's *Spinal Cord Injury (SCI) Facts and Figures* released in 2016,[1] there are approximately 17,000 new SCI cases each year in the United States. The annual incidence is approximately 54 cases per million population. During the past 40 years, there has been a significant change in the patterns of injury. Data show that the average age at the time of injury has increased from 29 years in the 1970s to approximately 42 years in the current decade. SCI cases are becoming more incomplete and older, approximately 80% of new SCI cases are men, and incomplete tetraplegia is the most frequent diagnosis.

Life expectancy for patients with SCI has improved with advancements in medical knowledge and management compared with life expectancy after World War II. However, unfortunately, there has been a plateau since the 1980s and it is still below the average years of life of a person without SCI. Mortality rates are higher during the first year after SCI, especially after high-level injuries and those requiring ventilator assistance.

The authors have nothing to disclose.
Department of Physical Medicine and Rehabilitation, McGovern Medical School, The University of Texas Health Science Center at Houston, 6431 Fannin Street, MSB G.550A, Houston, Texas 77030, USA
* Corresponding author.
E-mail address: joel.e.frontera@uth.tmc.edu

Phys Med Rehabil Clin N Am 28 (2017) 821–828
http://dx.doi.org/10.1016/j.pmr.2017.06.013
1047-9651/17/© 2017 Elsevier Inc. All rights reserved.

The National SCI database shows that pneumonia and septicemia have the greatest impact on decreased life expectancy in persons with SCI. Other factors, such as cancer, stroke, metabolic disorders, cardiovascular diseases, and mental disorders, also contribute to the mortality rates of this population.

This article covers some of the medical issues that affect SCI patients and discusses some of the day-to-day issues that face this patient population, such as quality of life (QoL), complications, and barriers for independence.

HEALTH COMPLICATIONS OF PERSONS WITH SPINAL CORD INJURY

As persons with SCI continue to age and as the average age of onset of SCI continues to trend older, multiple health complications are being noted by the medical professionals who work with this patient population.[2] On injury, a significant number of SCI patients develop issues with spasticity, weakness, and pain, as well as neurogenic bowel and bladder. Other issues now seen in a patient's medical history are osteoporosis,[3] pressure injuries, cardiovascular diseases,[4,5] and metabolic syndromes.[6-9] These issues have been shown to have a negative effect on QoL, social participation, and sex life.[10] The human body is expected to reach maximum functional status at approximately 25 years of age. This is the time that the major organ systems may reach peak functional capacity. After 25 years, this peak capacity tends to decrease at about 1% per year.[11] Immediately after SCI, the body accelerates its functional and metabolic decline; however, after the initial insult, the aging process continues at a normal rate. This may correlate with the findings that people that suffer SCI later in life may have poorer functional outcomes than those injured earlier in their life.[12]

CARDIOVASCULAR DISEASES

Even though pulmonary complications and infections are among the most common causes of death among persons with SCI, cardiovascular diseases are becoming increasingly common causes of premature death in this population. This is also associated with preventable risk factors such as smoking, decreased activity, and obesity.[13] The concern is that these preventable risk factors in combination with the underlying neurologic disorder may place this population at a greater risk for premature death than non-SCI persons.[14]

Multiple issues can affect the overall cardiovascular health in the long term. Some investigators note an accelerated risk for cardiovascular disorders that increases morbidity and mortality in SCI patients. The term cardiometabolic syndrome has been suggested to identify some of the effects post-SCI.[9] It has been shown that there is a significant decrease in cardioprotective high-density lipoprotein post-SCI. Dallmeijer and colleagues[15] have argued that this may be caused by post-SCI immobilization. Other causes include a poor diet and an increase in caloric content. Cardiometabolic syndrome also includes insulin resistance, obesity, and hypertension. The combination of all of these factors at the same time may have a profound effect on post-SCI health. Research continues to work on finding specific biomarkers for cardiovascular disease in SCI to guide medical evaluation and management.[16] Markers such as levels of C-reactive protein and plasma homocysteine, which have been shown to be predictors for increased atherogenesis and vascular disease, respectively, seem to be elevated in persons with SCI compared with non-SCI persons.[17-19]

MUSCULOSKELETAL CHANGES

Acute changes after SCI in muscle can predispose muscle to increase fatigability. Changes at the muscular level, such as increased atrophy, increased fat mass, and changes in the type of muscle fibers, tend to have a negative effect on strength, body mass index, and muscle mass. Even though there is a plateau in the first year or so after the injury, changes can continue to occur as the person ages.[8]

Changes in the upper extremity are also a known complication after SCI. Shoulder complications are a very common musculoskeletal complaint among persons with SCI (both paraplegic and tetraplegic). Persons with SCI put a significant strain on their shoulders for mobility and transfers. Depending on the neurologic level of injury, there may also be significant imbalance in the strength of different shoulder muscles. Studies have shown that persons with SCI tend to have increased degenerative changes in the glenohumeral joint compared with persons without SCI. These changes tend to progress and worsen as patients age.[20,21]

BONE HEALTH

Persons with SCI undergo significant bone loss in the first several weeks and months following their injuries.[22] During the first 4 months after injury, bone mineral density (BMD) loss has been reported to be as high as 27%. This is secondary to a significant demineralization process due to a marked osteoclastic activity. Other endocrine factors may also cause a premature onset of osteoporosis. The changes in the bone microarchitecture after SCI may lead to impaired calcium and vitamin-D metabolism.[23]

The distal femur and the proximal tibia seem to be the most affected areas. These sites are the most common areas of fractures from low-energy impact in persons with SCI.[24] These fractures have significant impact in the patient's QoL, functional independence, and overall health.

Treatment interventions have been controversial for chronic SCI. Bodyweight supported treadmill has been shown to be ineffective in preventing or reversing bone loss in patients.[25] On the other hand, the use of functional electrical stimulation cycle ergometry has been shown to have limited effectiveness in preserving BMD, especially in the distal femur and proximal tibia.[26–28] In terms of medical management, there is limited evidence regarding the effectiveness of multiple agents, such as bisphosphonates, in improving bone health. Future research should focus on suppression of osteoclastic activity and promotion of osteoblastic activity by multiple means.[22]

ENDOCRINE SYSTEM

Most of the evidence regarding changes in the endocrine system after SCI tends to be level 4 or 5. However, a significant part of this evidence shows that persons with SCI have decreased secretion of testosterone, as well as human growth hormone. This tends to happen prematurely in SCI patients and is hypothesized to cause advanced aging.

NEUROGENIC BLADDER

Urologic issues related to SCI have always been a major cause of morbidity and mortality among the SCI patient population. Multiple investigators[29–31] have reported that urologic issues are a major reason for health-related concerns and rehospitalization in patients with chronic SCI. Patients with neurogenic bladder usually manage their bladder with an intermittent catheterization program and indwelling catheter or suprapubic tube. More complex cases may require a surgical approach, such as a bladder augmentation surgery. This patient population is significantly at risk of developing complicated urinary tract infections (UTIs). It is expected that almost all patients will require antibiotic management of a UTI during their first year post-SCI. Other risks include urinary incontinence, bladder stones, kidney stones, and an increased risk of bladder cancer compared with the general population.

Some evidence points toward increased renal decline after years 4 and 5 postinjury. There is no specific evidence that suggests increased aging in this organ system. Even though they are predisposed to develop some conditions, as previously noted, good urologic follow-up and surveillance may help with complications in the long term. In terms of prostate issues, multiple studies have not shown an increase in prostate-specific antigen levels when compared with non-SCI subjects.[32]

PAIN

There is not a lot of information regarding the aging process of the central nervous system after SCI. The prevalence of pain after SCI is varied, ranging from 25% to greater than 90% of subjects, depending on the study. There does not seem to be a relationship between age of SCI, completeness of injury, or type of injury in regard to pain.[33] It has been shown that the development of neuropathic pain following SCI will most likely continue throughout the patient's life.[34] Most patients with neuropathic pain have no change in prevalence or intensity over time.[35] If there is an acute increase in neuropathic pain in a chronic SCI patient there should be a thorough evaluation of the causes of this increase. Management of chronic post-SCI pain should be done in the context of other common conditions affecting this specific patient population. Persons with SCI also may suffer from other disorders, such as depression, anxiety, cognitive impairments, spasticity, and other types of pain. The assessment should focus on identifying the type of pain (by using a pain classification method, such as the Bryce-Ragnarsson scale) and assessing for specific factors that may cause or exacerbate the condition.

MENTAL HEALTH

Mental health issues, such as depression and anxiety, are very common after SCI. An estimated 1 in 5 persons with SCI are diagnosed with depression[36] compared with approximately 16% of the general medical population in the United States. The prevalence of depression in SCI varies widely study to study. More studies are needed to accurately estimate the prevalence of depression in SCI so that measures are taken proactively to try to improve management. Possible risk factors that may predispose to an increased incidence of depression may include causes of injury, patient's demographics, and discharge disposition.[37] The causes for mental health issues, such as depression and anxiety, are still being debated. In the chronic SCI patient, other factors, such as decreased function and secondary medical complications, may have an increased role as the patient ages.

QUALITY OF LIFE AND PARTICIPATION

The struggle to maintain health and satisfaction with life throughout the aging process is a challenge faced by all human beings. Aging affects every organ system in the body and, from social life to work life to everything else, can profoundly change our lives. The interaction between aging and chronic SCI, itself a process that affects the whole body, produces special challenges for the affected individual and the medical professionals working to support them. However, these challenges should not be thought of as esoteric. In fact, SCI has been found to be a model for premature aging of various organ systems, including cardiovascular, musculoskeletal, and respiratory.[21] Aging patients with SCI experience a variety of symptoms that are not unknown to the unaffected aging population but may be more pronounced.[38] These symptoms in turn affect QoL and satisfaction with different aspects of life.[2,39,40] However, these challenges are not insurmountable.

As persons with SCI age, their independence in activities of daily living, such as dressing and toileting, decrease.[41] These declines in functional status are also noted in their exercise activities. Persons with SCI seem to not exercise or participate in social activities as much when they age.[2] These issues create a conundrum to the aging SCI population because it is well documented that exercise and physical activity can promote health and well-being.

The health complications experienced by aging individuals with SCI are wide ranging. They include fatigue, pain, increasing weakness, increasing risk for pressure sores, cardiovascular disease, and diabetes.[2] Bowel and bladder regulation problems may also develop. The frequency of most of these complications is increased with longer duration SCI.

In a study conducted in Stockholm, Sweden, 42% of participants with a prior SCI who responded to a survey reported problems such as pain, spasticity, weakness, and fatigue as the primary reasons for no longer engaging in active recreation. Also, 68% reported that the same symptoms were responsible for them no longer exercising. There was also a negative association between the use of a personal assistant and participation in exercise, which suggests that lack of independence also contributes to decreased participation. Other studies demonstrated that pain that interfered with daily activities was associated with declining self-reported QoL.[40,42]

Much like the general population, those with SCI experience fluctuations in their satisfaction with different aspects of their lives in relation to both their age and the time since their injury.[39,43,44] It is important for both clinicians and patients to realize that improvements in satisfaction with QoL in multiple domains and maintaining good to excellent satisfaction with QoL in the years following the injury are the rule rather than the exception. This has been demonstrated in multiple studies following patients out to 14 to 15 years postinjury.[45–48] Declines in satisfaction in some areas over time are to be expected. Persons with SCI were found to have a decrease in satisfaction with social life, sex life, and general health when measured 25 years postinjury.[10] However, this group was also found to have increased satisfaction with employment and satisfaction with their financial and living situations.

Aging persons with SCI, as well as clinicians, can draw several logical conclusions from these studies. The first is that more effort should be made to establish multidisciplinary medical clinics to address the multiple complications SCI patients may have that interfere with their daily lives and, therefore, their QoL. Additional research needs to be conducted to validate the effectiveness of this approach.[2,38] Because employment and personal independence seem to have beneficial effects on QoL as persons with SCI age, it could also be concluded that special effort should be made to maximize both of these in the early postinjury years of individuals with SCI. It should be emphasized that both aging and SCI are complex processes that affect every system of the human body and the interaction between these processes create special challenges for persons with SCI and the medical professionals who care for them. Although this is challenging, it is worth emphasizing that aging in the SCI population has important parallels to the general population, and scholarship and compassion for either can lead to finding these for the other.

SUMMARY

A few trends from the SCI research include

1. Older age of injury
2. Increased longevity
3. Increased incidence of secondary health complications
4. Perceived decrease in independence and physical activity with aging.

These trends point toward an apparent need for prevention and intervention in the acute phase of the injury. Screening patients for mental health issues, functional activities, QoL, and medical conditions in the immediate months after and SCI may help avoid some of the pitfalls of aging with and SCI. Even though persons with SCI have many issues to work on, their QoL has the potential to improve and even remain at higher levels. More data are needed to identify those factors that would make this happen.

REFERENCES

1. National Spinal Cord Injury Statistical Center. The University of Alabama at Birmingham Department of Physical Medicine and Rehabilitation. Facts and Figures at a Glance 2016. Available at: https://www.nscisc.uab.edu/Public/Facts%202016.pdf.
2. Lundström U, Wahman K, Seiger Å, et al. Participation in activities and secondary health complications among persons aging with traumatic spinal cord injury. Spinal Cord 2017;55(4):367–72.
3. Garland DE, Adkins RH, Rah A, et al. Bone loss with aging and the impact of SCI. Top Spinal Cord Inj Rehabil 2001;6:47–60.
4. Wahman K, Nash MS, Lewis JE, et al. Increased cardiovascular disease risk in Swedish persons with paraplegia: the Stockholm Spinal Cord Injury Study. J Rehabil Med 2010;42:489–92.
5. Jörgensen S, Iwarsson S, Norin L, et al. The Swedish Aging With Spinal Cord Injury Study (SASCIS): methodology and initial results. PM R 2016;8(7):667–77.
6. Lavela SL, Weaver FM, Goldstein B, et al. Diabetes mellitus in individuals with spinal cord injury or disorder. J Spinal Cord Med 2006;29:387–95.
7. Rajan S, McNeely MJ, Hammond M, et al. Association between obesity and diabetes mellitus in veterans with spinal cord injuries and disorders. Am J Phys Med Rehabil 2010;89:353–61.
8. Gorgey AS, Dolbow DR, Dolbow JD, et al. Effects of spinal cord injury on body composition and metabolic profile - part I. J Spinal Cord Med 2014 Nov;37(6): 693–702.
9. Nash MS, Tractenberg RE, Mendez AJ, et al. Cardiometabolic syndrome in people with spinal cord injury/disease: guideline-derived and nonguideline risk components in a pooled sample. Arch Phys Med Rehabil 2016;97(10):1696–705.
10. Krause J, Broderick L. A 25-year longitudinal study of the natural course of aging after spinal cord injury. Spinal Cord 2005;43:349–56.
11. Adkins RH. Research and interpretation perspectives on aging related physical morbidity with spinal cord injury and brief review of systems. NeuroRehabilitation 2004;19:3–13.
12. Furlan JC, Kattail D, Fehlings M. The impact of co-morbidities on age-related differences in mortality after acute traumatic spinal cord injury. J Neurotrauma 2009;26:1361–7.

13. Jensen MP, Truitt AR, Schomer KG, et al. Frequency and age effects of secondary health conditions in individuals with spinal cord injury: a scoping review. Spinal Cord 2013;51:882–92.
14. Garshick E, Kelley A, Cohen S, et al. A prospective assessment of mortality in chronic spinal cord injury. Spinal Cord 2005;43:408–16.
15. Dallmeijer AJ, van der Woude LH, van Kamp GJ, et al. Changes in lipid, lipoprotein and apolipoprotein profiles in persons with spinal cord injuries during the first 2 years post-injury. Spinal Cord 1999;37:96–102.
16. Nash M, Dalal K, Martinez-Barrizonte J, et al. Suppression of proatherogenic inflammatory cytokines as a therapeutic countermeasure to CVD risks accompanying SCI. Top Spinal Cord Inj Rehabil 2010;16:14–32.
17. Bauman WA, Adkins RH, Spungen AM, et al. Levels of plasma homocysteine in persons with spinal cord injury. J Spinal Cord Med 2001;24:81–6.
18. Wang TD, Wang YH, Hung TS, et al. Circulating levels of markers of inflammation and endothelial activation are increased in men with chronic spinal cord injury. J Formos Med Assoc 2007;106:919–28.
19. Tsitouras PD, Zhong YG, Spungen AM, et al. Serum testosterone and growth hormone/insulin-like growth factor-I in adults with spinal cord injury. Horm Metab Res 1995;27:287–92.
20. Kivimäki J, Ahoniemi E. Ultrasonographic findings in shoulders of able-bodied, paraplegic and tetraplegic subjects. Spinal Cord 2008;46:50–2.
21. Hitzig S, Eng J, Miller W, et al. An evidence-based review of aging of the body systems following spinal cord injury. Spinal Cord 2011;49(6):684–701.
22. Cirnigliaro CM, Myslinski MJ, La Fountaine MF, et al. Bone loss at the distal femur and proximal tibia in persons with spinal cord injury: imaging approaches, risk of fracture, and potential treatment options. Osteoporos Int 2017;28:747.
23. Eser P, Frotzler A, Zehnder Y, et al. Relationship between the duration of paralysis and bone structure: a pQCT study of spinal cord injured individuals. Bone 2004; 34:869–80.
24. Morse LR, Battaglino RA, Stolzmann KL, et al. Osteoporotic fractures and hospitalization risk in chronic spinal cord injury. Osteoporos Int 2009;20(3):385–92.
25. Giangregorio LM, Hicks AL, Webber CE, et al. Body weight supported treadmill training in acute spinal cord injury: impact on muscle and bone. Spinal Cord 2005;43(11):649–57.
26. Bloomfield SA, Mysiw WJ, Jackson RD. Bone mass and endocrine adaptations to training in spinal cord injured individuals. Bone 1996;19(1):61–8.
27. Eser P, de Bruin ED, Telley I, et al. Effect of electrical stimulation-induced cycling on bone mineral density in spinal cord-injured patients. Eur J Clin Invest 2003; 33(5):412–9.
28. Lai CH, Chang WH, Chan WP, et al. Effects of functional electrical stimulation cycling exercise on bone mineral density loss in the early stages of spinal cord injury. J Rehabil Med 2010;42(2):150–4.
29. Bloemen-Vrencken JHA, Post MWM, Hendriks JMS, et al. Health problems of persons with spinal cord injury living in the Netherlands. Disabil Rehabil 2005;27: 1381–9.
30. Klotz R, Joseph PA, Ravaud JF, et al. The Tetrafigap Survey on the long-term outcome of tetraplegia spinal cord injured persons: Part III. Medical complications and associated factors. Spinal Cord 2002;40:457–67.
31. Adriaansen JJ, Ruijs LE, van Koppenhagen CF, et al. Secondary health conditions and quality of life in persons living with spinal cord injury for at least ten years. J Rehabil Med 2016;48(10):853–60.

32. Shim HB, Kim YD, Jung TY, et al. Prostate-specific antigen and prostate volume in Korean men with spinal cord injury: a case-control study. Spinal Cord 2008; 46(1):11.
33. Saulino M. Spinal cord injury pain. Phys Med Rehabil Clin N Am 2014;25(2): 397–410.
34. Siddall PJ, McClelland JM, Rutkowski SB, et al. A longitudinal study of the prevalence and characteristics of pain in the first 5 years following spinal cord injury. Pain 2003;103:249–57.
35. Jensen MP, Hoffman AJ, Cardenas DD. Chronic pain in individuals with spinal cord injury: A survey and longitudinal study. Spinal Cord 2005;43:704–12.
36. Williams R, Adrian Murray MA. Prevalence of depression after spinal cord injury: a meta-analysis. Arch Phys Med Rehabil 2015;96:133–40.
37. Lim S-W, Shiue Y-L, Ho C-H, et al. Anxiety and depression in patients with traumatic spinal cord injury: a nationwide population-based cohort study. PLoS One 2017;12(1):e0169623.
38. Molton IR, Terrill AL, Smith AE, et al. Modeling secondary health conditions in adults aging with physical disability. J Aging Health 2014;26(3):335–59.
39. Savic G, Charlifue S, Glass C, et al. British Ageing with SCI study: changes in physical and psychological outcomes over time. Top Spinal Cord Inj Rehabil 2010;15(3):41–53.
40. Putzke JD, Richards JS, Hicken BL, et al. Interference due to pain following spinal cord injury: important predictors and impact on quality of life. Pain 2002;100(3): 231–42.
41. Liem N, McColl M, King W, et al. Aging with a spinal cord injury: factors associated with the need for more help with activities of daily living. Arch Phys Med Rehabil 2004;85:1567–77.
42. Stensman R. Adjustment to traumatic spinal cord injury: a longitudinal study of self-reported quality of life. Paraplegia 1994;32(6):416–22.
43. Sakakibara BM, Hitzig SL, Miller WC, et al. An evidence-based review on the influence of aging with a spinal cord injury on subjective quality of life. Spinal Cord 2012;50(8):570–8.
44. Kunzmann U, Little TD, Smith J. Is age-related stability of subjective well-being a paradox? Cross-sectional and longitudinal evidence from the Berlin Aging Study. Psychol Aging 2000;15(3):511–26.
45. Chen Y, Anderson CJ, Vogel LC, et al. Change in life satisfaction of adults with pediatric-onset spinal cord injury. Arch Phys Med Rehabil 2008;89(12):2285–92.
46. Bushnik T. Access to equipment, participation, and quality of life in aging individuals with high tetraplegia. Top Spinal Cord Inj Rehabil 2002;7(3):17–27.
47. Bushnik T, Charlifue S. Longitudinal study of individuals with high tetraplegia (C1–C4) 14 to 24 years postinjury. Top Spinal Cord Inj Rehabil 2005;10(3):79–93.
48. Krause JS, Coker JL. Aging after spinal cord injury: a 30-year longitudinal study. J Spinal Med 2006;29(4):371–6.

Rehabilitation Needs of the Elder with Traumatic Brain Injury

Manuel F. Mas, MD[a],*, Amy Mathews, MD[b],
Ekua Gilbert-Baffoe, MD[b]

KEYWORDS

• Traumatic brain injury • Elderly • Cognitive rehabilitation • Preventive medicine

KEY POINTS

• As the US population ages, the number of adults aging with a traumatic brain injury (TBI) and elderly patients with new TBIs will increase.
• Falls are the leading cause of TBI in adults over the age of 65.
• The needs of elderly patients with TBI are unique.
• Acute inpatient rehabilitation programs should be individualized and include interventions to address cognitive dysfunction, motor recovery, and preventive medicine.
• Elderly patients make meaningful functional gains during inpatient rehabilitation, with high rates of home discharges. These gains may be realized over longer durations of stay.

INTRODUCTION

Traumatic brain injury (TBI) is one of the leading causes of chronic disability in the United States.[1] A TBI occurs when an external force causes an alternation in brain function and/or other evidence of brain pathology.[1] TBI is often referred to as a "silent epidemic," owing to limited public awareness and to the associated complications, such as cognitive dysfunction, that may not be readily apparent.[2] A TBI has adverse effects not only on the individual, but their family, and the local and global economy.[3]

Recent studies suggest a prevalence of TBI, in the general population, of 12% to 16.7% in males and 8.5% in females.[4] In the United States, approximately 1.7 million people sustain a TBI annually.[2] A trimodal age distribution of injury risk demonstrates

Disclosure: The authors have nothing to disclose.
[a] Department of Physical Medicine and Rehabilitation, McGovern Medical School, The University of Texas Health Science Center at Houston, TIRR Memorial Hermann, 1333 Moursund Street, Houston, TX 77030, USA; [b] Department of Physical Medicine and Rehabilitation, Baylor College of Medicine, 7200 Cambridge Street, Suite 10C, Houston, TX 77030, USA
* Corresponding author.
E-mail address: manuel.mas@uth.tmc.edu

that individuals under the age of 5, individuals between the ages of 15 and 24, and adults over the age of 65 are at an increased risk for sustaining a TBI.[5] Adults aged 75 years and older have the highest rates of TBI-related hospitalization and death.[2] The rate of TBI-related hospitalizations in patients 65 years and older is estimated at 155.9 per 100,000. This rate increases dramatically with advancing age reaching 366.6 per 100,000 for patients 85 years and older.[6]

Falls are the leading cause of TBI in adults over the age of 65. From 2002 to 2010, there was an increase in fall-related TBIs, hospitalizations, and TBI-related deaths among adults aged 65 and older.[2] In this group, the estimated rate of TBI-related hospitalizations owing to a fall is 104.9 per 100,00. Fall-related TBI hospitalization increases with age, reaching 6 times this rate in those 85 years and older.[6]

With an increasing general life expectancy, both the prevalence of people living with TBI and the rates of incident TBI in the elderly are expected to increase.[7] In this context, there is a growing need to understand the effects of TBI on the aging population. Physiatrists treating this patient population should be aware of the unique rehabilitation needs of the elder patient in the acute rehabilitation setting, the interactions between TBI and advanced age, and the prognostic implications of TBI in an elderly population.

THE CONTINUUM OF REHABILITATION AFTER TRAUMATIC BRAIN INJURY IN THE ELDERLY
Acute Care

Rehabilitation for any individual who experiences a TBI begins in the acute care setting. Although the focus of care during this stage is on the prevention of secondary brain injury, rehabilitation after a TBI is ideally initiated while the patient resides in the intensive care setting.[8] In fact, the presence of a physiatrist involved in the care of the patient during this early stage has been associated with improved functional outcomes.[9] Here, the goal is prevention of complications secondary to prolonged immobilization, including skin breakdown and joint contractures. When compared with their younger counterparts, older individuals who suffer a TBI possess more comorbidities that can affect their rehabilitation care. Among these, cardiopulmonary compromise and an increased prevalence of osteoarthritis can affect the precautions and interventions provided by therapists, not only during this acute stage but throughout the entire rehabilitation spectrum.

Inpatient Rehabilitation

Inpatient rehabilitation can be a viable alternative for elderly patients with a TBI once stabilized and discharged from the acute care setting. They must meet the same admission criteria as any other patient before acceptance to an inpatient rehabilitation facility, including the need for constant medical and nursing supervision and deficits requiring at least 3 hours of therapy. The rehabilitation team must be vigilant of several comorbidities when following this population in an inpatient rehabilitation facility.

Polypharmacy
Polypharmacy and the concurrent use of psychotropic medications is common in TBI patients during postacute rehabilitation.[10] In fact, psychotropic medication administration generally increases during the course of inpatient rehabilitation for TBI.[11] Commonly prescribed psychotropic drugs include anticonvulsants, antidepressants, antipsychotics, anxiolytics, stimulants, and hypnotics.[10,11] Additionally, other classes of medications such as proton pump inhibitors, antithrombotic agents, beta-blockers, and antihypertensive agents are prevalent in TBI patients during rehabilitation and can

have a potential functional impact.[10] Off-label use of psychotropic medications in the postacute care of TBI patients is common, primarily for agitation, behavioral disturbances, insomnia, and pain.[12] Polypharmacy has been associated with severe impairment and age, more so with patients older than 65 years of age.[10,11] Polypharmacy is also commonly observed in the older community-dwelling population and has been linked to frailty in this group.[13,14]

Polypharmacy has been linked to worse outcomes during rehabilitation.[15] Polypharmacy in patients with a TBI has been associated with falls, which in itself is the primary cause of TBI in the elderly.[16] Yet, polypharmacy may be appropriately driven by multimorbidity, particularly in elderly TBI patients. Surveillance of drug–drug interactions and medication safety is imperative to reduce polypharmacy in this population and increase the likelihood of better outcomes.

Posttraumatic hydrocephalus

Posttraumatic hydrocephalus (PTH) is a serious and treatable complication after TBI. This sequelae is classically defined as a distention in the ventricular system within the brain owing to inadequate passage of cerebrospinal fluid (CSF).[17] Its incidence has been estimated to range from 8% to 45% within 1 year of injury.[18–20] It is more likely to occur during inpatient rehabilitation, limiting progress, prolonging stay, and negatively affecting outcomes.[20] PTH after TBI has been significantly associated with older age, presence of traumatic subarachnoid hemorrhage, and a history of decompressive cranial surgery.[18,20] It has been postulated that excessive subarachnoid fibrosis after TBI in older patients can lead to impaired CSF circulation and decreased reabsorption.[21] Thus, physiatrists managing elderly patients with a TBI must be vigilant of this complication. Many of the classically described signs of PTH, including ataxia, dementia, and urinary incontinence, overlap with the classic triad of normal pressure hydrocephalus. Although these classic symptoms may be present in patients with PTH, they may be misattributed to primary brain injury effects, including alterations in consciousness, severe mobility impairments, and neurogenic bladder. Thus, a halt or regression in progress during inpatient rehabilitation may be a more appropriate sign of PTH in a TBI patient. At this time, there are no established diagnostic criteria for PTH after TBI[22]; therefore, clinicians following elderly TBI patients must maintain a high suspicion for PTH to pursue further diagnostic workup, including obtaining imaging studies. Identifying PTH on imaging can be particularly challenging in older patients with cerebral atrophy where it is difficult to distinguish ex vacuo ventricular dilation from abnormalities in CSF flow dynamics secondary to CSF malabsorption or obstruction.[23] PTH requires diversion of CSF, usually by means of a ventriculostomy drain, such as a ventriculoperitoneal shunt. Earlier ventricular shunting is associated with improved recovery.[19]

Cognitive impairment

Older individuals can experience a cognitive decline over their life span owing to normal aging. In most patients, normal aging does not cause a notable deterioration in functional abilities, but some may experience mild cognitive impairment, where impaired function does not yet meet criteria for dementia.[24] Others may progress from mild cognitive impairment to dementia. It is known that elderly people with cognitive impairments are at an increased risk of TBI and that this cohort can have particularly poor functional outcomes owing to their decreased premorbid cognitive reserve.[8]

Beyond cognitive changes associated with normal aging or preinjury dementia, elderly patients may experience additional neuropsychiatric sequelae after a TBI, including deterioration in cognitive domains such as intelligence, attention, executive functions, and memory.[25] When evaluating the neuropsychological profile in older adults, those with a TBI had greater deficits in processing speed and executive functioning.[26] The underdiagnoses of preinjury cognitive impairment[27] in the elderly complicates the evaluation and management of cognition in older patients after TBI because it is more difficult to identify true cognitive decline from baseline. Ideally, clinicians should be aware of the patient's premorbid cognitive status to establish realistic goals and appropriate therapeutic interventions.

A neuropsychiatric evaluation is essential when evaluating cognitive domains in the elder TBI patient and should precede any interventions targeted at cognitive enhancement.[28] There is strong evidence for the use of cognitive rehabilitation interventions for attention, memory, social communication skills, executive function, and comprehensive–holistic neuropsychological rehabilitation, which includes individual and group therapy emphasizing metacognitive and emotional regulation.[29] Physical exercise has also been linked to cognitive recovery after TBI.[30] Thus, nonpharmacologic interventions for cognitive rehabilitation should precede pharmacologic options. Pharmacologic options should only be used adjunctively to other interventions. Proper selection of pharmacotherapy warrants consideration of the injury severity and time frame and intended treatment target, among other factors. Catecholamine and cholinergic augmenters as well as glutamatergic stabilizers are generally used in treating posttraumatic cognitive impairments.[31] Clinicians must be vigilant of the risk of polypharmacy and poor outcomes in the older TBI patient (as detailed) when selecting pharmacologic interventions for cognitive deficits.

Behavioral and affective disturbance

Like cognitive decline, emotional changes are common in both older adults and those who experience a TBI. In both cases, depressive disorders are the most prevalent mental health problems and are often underreported by the elderly.[32,33] Depression can negatively affect outcomes after geriatric inpatient rehabilitation, even to a greater extent than impaired cognition, increased pain, and low education.[34] Thus, the diagnosis and management of depression in an older adult with a TBI must be timely to allow for optimal outcomes after inpatient rehabilitation. Identifying depression in the elderly patient with a TBI can prove difficult owing to presence of comorbid conditions and underreporting of symptoms. The effects of TBI can also mask or mimic symptoms of depression. Because patient with a TBI can demonstrate apathy, cognitive deterioration, fatigue, and somatic symptoms, clinicians must carefully evaluate these symptoms before attributing them to the mechanism of injury rather than to a primary mood disturbance.[8] Other behavioral problems that can be encountered in this population include mania, anxiety, apathy, agitation, aggression, and pathologic laughing and crying.

Nonpharmacologic interventions should be used initially to manage behavioral and affective disturbances. These interventions can include identification and modification of triggers, group therapy, behavioral therapy, and psychotherapy, with psychotherapy being the preferred treatment option for older patients suffering from depression.[35] These interventions should be individualized based on symptomatology and other comorbid factors. An integrated approach focusing on personal participation goals has been proven to decrease symptoms of depression up to a year after stroke in an older adult cohort.[36] Pharmacotherapy can be a viable adjuvant in the management of behavioral and affective disorders in this population. Selective serotonin reuptake inhibitors are well-tolerated and evidenced for the treatment of depression after a TBI.[37] Selective serotonin reuptake inhibitors are useful to treat other affective disturbances, such as anxiety, aggression, and pathologic laughing and crying.[38] Methylphenidate can be used as a rapid treatment alternative for depression in the inpatient setting.[39] However, the clinician must carefully evaluate every new medication and its potential side effects in the elderly patient with a TBI before its prescription. Atypical antipsychotics have been linked with increased mortality.[40] Benzodiazepines and typical antipsychotics can impair recovery after TBI and are typically not recommended.[40] Tricyclic antidepressants can cause cardiac and cognitive abnormalities in the elderly owing to their anticholinergic properties. Nortriptyline is preferred over other tricyclic antidepressants owing to their preferable safety profile in the elderly. As with cognitive impairments, the clinician should avoid polypharmacy and incorporate a holistic approach to the rehabilitation plan, focusing on nonpharmacologic interventions with medications serving only as adjuvants to decrease symptom burden.

Orthostatic hypotension

Orthostatic hypotension is common in the elderly.[41] It is defined as a decrease of 20 mm Hg in the systolic blood pressure and/or decrease of 10 mm Hg in the diastolic blood pressure within 3 minutes of sitting or standing.[42] Common symptoms include dizziness or lightheadedness with standing, blurry vision, weakness, or confusion. Orthostatic hypotension is often cited as a risk factor for falls in older adults.[43] Orthostatic hypotension has also been associated with poor global cognitive function, poor memory, and worse prognosis in elderly patients with dementia.[44,45] Elderly patients with a TBI may experience orthostatic hypotension with functional training during their stay and may require closer monitoring of their vitals and symptoms. These patients benefit from slower positional transitions during transfers and ambulation, allowing more time for cardiovascular habituation to postural changes. A careful evaluation of the patient's drug regimen is warranted to modify or avoid potential contributors, including dopaminergic agents (ie, amantadine, bromocriptine, carbidopa-levodopa), diuretics, and overprescription of antihypertensive medications. Abdominal binders and compression stockings may aid elderly patients with a TBI with orthostatic hypotension. Finally, agents such as midodrine and fludrocortisone may be used when other interventions are ineffective.

Additional considerations

There are additional aspects inherent to this population that must be considered during inpatient rehabilitation. Clinicians should be vigilant of premorbid visual and auditory deficits that may be confounded or exacerbated by a TBI and may require modifications of therapeutic interventions. Sleep disturbances and fatigue are prevalent with advanced age and after a TBI. The evaluation and management of these deficits can potentially improve outcomes during inpatient rehabilitation stay. As with other symptomatology, avoiding polypharmacy is imperative. Last, as with any patient suffering from a TBI, older adults are also at risk of developing neurogenic bladder and bowel, spasticity, pain, and headaches, which must be addressed during their rehabilitation stay.

Functional Outcomes

After the implementation of the Medicare Prospective Payment System, there has been increasing pressure on inpatient rehabilitation facilities to identify patients who will achieve sufficient functional gains in a manner that efficiently uses limited rehabilitation and health care resources.[46,47] The framework of the Prospective Payment System becomes especially relevant in the consideration of the elderly TBI population, because they represent a unique cohort with potentially different rehabilitation needs. Multiple studies have demonstrated that elderly patients benefit from acute inpatient rehabilitation and make significant changes in mean Functional Independence

Measure (FIM) and Disability Rating Scale (DRS) scores.[47–49] These improvements, compared with younger patients, occur over longer durations of stay, which contribute to lower FIM efficiencies, slower rates of improvement on the DRS, and greater total inpatient rehabilitation charges.[47,48,50] Potential explanations for these differences are that elderly patients have lower physical and cognitive reserve, a higher incidence of medical complications and comorbidities, more cognitive impairments that prevent new learning, and less efficient neuroplasticity.[48,51–54]

Despite these obstacles, elderly patients with TBI can be discharged to the community.[48] There are conflicting data regarding disposition outcomes compared with younger TBI populations; however, some studies report lower community discharge rates and greater dependence compared with younger patients.[6,47,49] Risk factors for institutionalization after inpatient rehabilitation include older age at time of injury, living alone before TBI, duration of posttraumatic amnesia, and lower discharge FIM scores for locomotion, bed–chair–toilet transfers, and social interaction.[55] Few studies have reported similar disposition outcomes for elderly patients compared with younger patients,[48,50] and these controlled for a variety of demographic and injury-related factors.

Studies on functional and disposition outcomes of the elderly with TBI must be interpreted with methodological limitations in mind. Much of the studies report on relatively short-term outcomes on the order of weeks to months, but functional gains may be achieved with time beyond what is captured in the data sets.[47,48] Age groupings must be considered, because some studies group patients greater than 55 years into the "elderly" category and others use definitions of greater than 65 years or greater than 75 years; in reality, these age groups may each have different needs and outcomes.[48,50] Most studies did not control for intensity or type of therapy, which may be geared to simpler or less aggressive protocols in the elderly. Additionally, most studies did not incorporate factors, such as comorbid medical conditions, premorbid functional status, or payer source, into their analysis and these factors may impact functional outcomes and durations of stay.

After acute inpatient rehabilitation, long-term outcomes after TBI are also impacted by age. Older patients show greater decline in functional and cognitive FIM, DRS, and cognitive scores with increasing time after injury.[56,57] This is not to say that elderly patients will consistently and steadily decline after inpatient rehabilitation. Advancing age was associated with improvement in expression and comprehension 1 to 5 years after injury. Additionally, age was not associated with changes in the FIM scores for memory, problem solving, or social interaction.[58]

Community integration, which encompasses meaningful and productive social, community, and in-home participation, becomes more difficult with advancing age.[59] Older people tend to have poorer community integration outcomes compared with younger patients with TBI with regard to several factors, including driving, shopping, money management, employment, and social engagement.[60–62] Rapport and colleagues,[63] however, report that the ability to drive is more predictive of successful community integration, rather than age. A dearth of community services, difficulty accessing transportation, attitudes of society and caregivers, and physical barriers in the environment have been identified as extrinsic factors that may impede community integration. Intrinsic factors to elderly patients with a TBI that contribute to participation restrictions include comorbidities that decrease community participation, challenging behaviors, and level of disability.[64–66]

Psychiatric sequelae must also be considered in discussion of long-term outcomes and community integration because they affect quality of life and community reentry. In the first decade after a TBI, rates of depression and anxiety are more common than in the uninjured, community-dwelling population. Advancing age, however, has not been found to be associated with higher rates of psychiatric morbidity in patients after TBI.[67] Despite this, depression after TBI in the elderly must be promptly and effectively addressed because it has been associated with worse global outcomes as well as lower scores on measures of working memory, processing speed, and executive functioning.[68]

In conclusion, elderly patients make meaningful functional gains with rehabilitation, but these improvements may take more time. Additionally, the rehabilitation needs of elderly patients may persist for longer after inpatient discharge. Ultimately, more studies are needed to identify the subset of elderly patients who will respond most effectively to inpatient rehabilitation, but also to identify patients in which to expect longer recovery courses. Further resources need to be developed to meet the needs of this population that may require an increased amount or duration of rehabilitation services.

Aging with a Traumatic Brain Injury

Through the aging process, the noninjured brain undergoes several structural and functional changes. With advancing age, the volume of the cerebral cortex, most notably the frontal gray matter, decreases. This process is postulated to be one of the mechanisms that contributes to decline in cognitive abilities with age.[69] After a TBI, the cerebral structure is often altered in the frontal and temporal lobes, owing to the bony floor of the skull. This affects a wide array of cognitive networks and leads to a myriad of neuropsychiatric and functional effects.[70] The overlay of TBI on an aging brain, however, is less well-understood. This interaction between aging and TBI becomes particularly important in the process of setting clinical expectations with patients and families, prognosticating, counseling, and designing research studies.[71]

Beyond the acute and subacute phases after brain injury, relatively little is understood regarding the long-term evolution of symptoms after TBI. Investigations into the process of aging with a TBI have mainly been cross-sectional and have shown that patients continue to change many years after their initial injury.[72,73] Thus, there has been a shift in viewpoint so that TBI should not be viewed as an isolated event but rather a long-term condition with a traumatic event representing the initiation of a dynamic disease process. The occurrence of a TBI in a patient's life can influence the aging process by introducing acute symptoms that persist through life, precipitating the premature onset of "age-related" cognitive decline, and contributing to the development of neurodegenerative diseases.

Cognitive and neuropsychiatric symptoms that occur acutely after TBI may be sustained through late adulthood. In a cohort study, reportedly asymptomatic middle-aged and elderly patients who sustained a mild or moderate TBI routinely performed inferiorly to age-matched healthy controls on tasks of memory and performance speed. Middle-aged patients with a TBI performed similarly to elderly subjects with a TBI, suggesting that a TBI sustained early in life may mimic cognitive changes typically attributed to age.[74] Although symptom persistence and pervasiveness may vary per several factors, including demographics, genetics, and injury characteristics, even seemingly asymptomatic patients may be experiencing persistent cognitive sequela.

It has also been postulated that TBI-related changes may contribute to the earlier or exacerbated onset of "normal," age-related changes. The microglial priming theory suggested by Ziebell and colleagues,[75] proposes that, after a TBI, microglial cells may maintain a proinflammatory profile. This state of glial dysfunction influences neuroplastic processes such as recovery from subsequent TBIs and aging so that, after a

TBI, the brain may have less effective regenerative and restorative capacities for the aging process.

TBI may influence the aging process by contributing to the development of neurodegenerative processes. This relationship is debated with some studies demonstrating little association between TBI and dementia or Alzheimer's disease[76] and other studies revealing accelerated or increased risk of dementia after TBI,[77–79] including some studies that showed exacerbated onset of Alzheimer's disease.[80,81]

Neuropathologically, patients who have sustained a TBI acutely demonstrate greater amounts of amyloid beta plaques,[82] which are hallmarks of many neurodegenerative diseases. From these studies, it was suggested that head trauma can increase susceptibility to neurodegenerative processes such as Alzheimer's disease.[83] The apolipoprotein E gene, namely the $\epsilon 4$ allele, has been shown to be related to both development of sporadic Alzheimer's disease and deposition of beta-amyloid protein

---

Box 1
A comprehensive rehabilitation plan for the elderly patient with a traumatic brain injury

Prevention
- Minimize fall risk factors
- Reduce polypharmacy

Inpatient rehabilitation
- Avoid polypharmacy
- Maintain vigilance for posttraumatic hydrocephalus
- Treat orthostatic hypotension
- Optimize sleep–wake cycles
- Assess auditory dysfunction
- Assess visual deficits
- Evaluate and treat cognitive deficits
- Assess for behavioral and affective disturbances
- Evaluate and treat for nociceptive and neuropathic pain
- Manage neurogenic bladder and bowel, when present
- Address headaches
- Evaluate and manage spasticity

Long-term interventions
- Fall risk prevention
  - Muscle activity, balance enhancement (eg, Tai Chi[6])
  - Avoid polypharmacy
- Maintain general medical health, including bone health
- Continued evaluation for neuropsychiatric, behavioral, and affective disorders.
- Screen for caregiver burnout and offer support resources if needed
- Assist with community reintegration strategies
- Encourage aerobic activity to maintain cardiovascular health
- Reassess need for further therapy participation
- Medical assessment for driving screening

after a head injury.[84] This idea supports the concept that the APO∈ 4 allele may confer a genetic susceptibility that, when accompanied by head trauma, may predispose the patient to neurodegenerative disorders with aging.[83] From a functional standpoint, patients with a brain injury who possess the APOE ∈4 have been shown to have decreased cognitive[85,86] and functional[87,88] gains after rehabilitation.

Life Expectancy

In an era of individualization of health care, it seems to be increasingly essential that physicians be able to delineate the factors that will affect an individuals' survival. Despite rehabilitative goals for functional outcome, several studies demonstrate the association of age and severity of functional disability as significant predictors of survival rates.[89]

Life expectancy after a TBI is reduced, on average, by 9 years with older age being an independent risk factor for death. Older age groups have an increased number of risk factors associated to death when compared with their younger counterparts. These factors include age, sex, marital status, mechanism of injury, FIM Motor subscale at discharge, and DRS score at discharge. Generally, an increase in age and DRS score at discharge suggests increased risk of death. Female sex and single status seem to be protective factors. Finally, falls and low FIM scores at discharge place individuals at a higher risk of death. Additionally, cause of death in the elder population with TBI seems to be more directly related to the level of debility.[90]

A Comprehensive Rehabilitation Plan

Older adults have an increased risk of sustaining a TBI. Physiatrists can play a crucial role in the acute rehabilitation after a TBI as well as in the long-term care of these patients, including the prevention of new injuries. A comprehensive neurorehabilitation plan should address cognitive dysfunction, motor recovery, and preventive medicine. However, with an understanding that TBI in the elderly confer unique characteristics, a more individualized plan can be formulated by the medical team[91] (**Box 1**). For the elderly population, this not only includes a focus on motor recovery and rehabilitation, but also a focus on the management of chronic and acute medical conditions and incorporation of risk-stratified care management.

REFERENCES

1. Frieden TR, Houry D, Baldwin G. Traumatic brain injury in the United States: epidemiology and rehabilitation. CDC NIH Rep to Congr 2015;1–74. http://dx.doi.org/10.3171/2009.10.JNS091500.

2. Faul M, Xu L, Wald MM, et al. Traumatic brain injury in the United States: emergency department visits, hospitalizations, and deaths. Centers Dis Control Prev Natl Cent Inj Prev Control 2010;891–904. http://dx.doi.org/10.1016/B978-0-444-52910-7.00011-8.

3. Albrecht JS, Slejko JF, Stein DM, et al. Treatment charges for traumatic brain injury among older adults at a trauma center. J Head Trauma Rehabil 2017;1. http://dx.doi.org/10.1097/HTR.0000000000000297.

4. Frost RB, Farrer TJ, Primosch M, et al. Prevalence of traumatic brain injury in the general adult population: a meta-analysis. Neuroepidemiology 2013;40(3):154–9.

5. Ramanathan DM, McWilliams N, Schatz P, et al. Epidemiological shifts in elderly traumatic brain injury: 18-year trends in Pennsylvania. J Neurotrauma 2012;29(7): 1371–8.

6. Coronado VG, Thomas KE, Sattin RW, et al. The CDC traumatic brain injury surveillance system: characteristics of persons aged 65 years and older hospitalized with a TBI. J Head Trauma Rehabil 2005;20(3):215–28.

7. Hoyert DL. 75 years of mortality in the United States, 1935-2010. NCHS Data Brief 2012;(88):1–8.

8. Levine J, Flanagan S. Traumatic brain injury in the elderly. In: Zasler ND, Katz DI, Zafonte RD, editors. Brain injury medicine, 2nd edition. Principles and practice. 2013. p. 420–33.

9. Greiss C, Yonclas PP, Jasey N, et al. Presence of a dedicated trauma center physiatrist improves functional outcomes following traumatic brain injury. J Trauma Acute Care Surg 2016;80(1):70–5.

10. Cosano G, Giangreco M, Ussai S, et al. Polypharmacy and the use of medications in inpatients with acquired brain injury during post-acute rehabilitation: a cross-sectional study. Brain Inj 2016;30(3):353–62.

11. Hammond FM, Barrett RS, Shea T, et al. Psychotropic medication use during inpatient rehabilitation for traumatic brain injury. Arch Phys Med Rehabil 2015; 96(8):S256–73.

12. Pisa FE, Cosano G, Giangreco M, et al. Prescribing practice and off-label use of psychotropic medications in post-acute brain injury rehabilitation centres: a cross-sectional survey. Brain Inj 2015;29(4):508–16.

13. Saum KU, Schöttker B, Meid AD, et al. Is polypharmacy associated with frailty in older people? Results from the ESTHER cohort study. J Am Geriatr Soc 2017b; 65(2):e27–32.

14. Husson N, Watfa G, Laurain M-C, et al. Characteristics of polymedicated ($\geq$ 4) elderly: a survey in a community-dwelling population aged 60 years and over. J Nutr Health Aging 2014;18(1):87–91.

15. Kose E, Maruyama R, Okazoe S, et al. Impact of polypharmacy on the rehabilitation outcome of Japanese stroke patients in the convalescent rehabilitation ward. J Aging Res 2016;2016:1–8.

16. Murphy MP, Carmine H, Kolakowsky-Hayner S. Modifiable and nonmodifiable risk factors for falls after traumatic brain injury: an exploratory investigation with implications for medication use. Rehabil Nurs 2014;39(3):113–22.

17. Rekate HL, Pudenz RH, Nulsen FE, et al. A contemporary definition and classification of hydrocephalus. Semin Pediatr Neurol 2009;16(1):9–15.

18. Mazzini L, Campini R, Angelino E, et al. Posttraumatic hydrocephalus: a clinical, neuroradiologic, and neuropsychologic assessment of long-term outcome. Arch Phys Med Rehabil 2003;84(11):1637–41. Available at: http://www.ncbi.nlm.nih.gov/pubmed/14639563. Accessed January 28, 2017.

19. Weintraub AH, Gerber DJ, Kowalski RG. Posttraumatic hydrocephalus as a confounding influence on brain injury rehabilitation: incidence, clinical characteristics, and outcomes. Arch Phys Med Rehabil 2017;98(2):312–9.

20. Kammersgaard LP, Linnemann M, Tibæk M. Hydrocephalus following severe traumatic brain injury in adults. Incidence, timing, and clinical predictors during rehabilitation. NeuroRehabilitation 2013;33(3):473–80.

21. Tian H-L, Xu T, Hu J, et al. Risk factors related to hydrocephalus after traumatic subarachnoid hemorrhage. Surg Neurol 2008;69(3):241–6.

22. Guyot LL, Michael DB. Post-traumatic hydrocephalus. Neurol Res 2000;22(1): 25–8. Available at: http://www.ncbi.nlm.nih.gov/pubmed/10672577. Accessed January 28, 2017.

23. Marmarou A, Foda MA, Bandoh K, et al. Posttraumatic ventriculomegaly: hydrocephalus or atrophy? A new approach for diagnosis using CSF dynamics. J Neurosurg 1996;85(6):1026–35.
24. Petersen RC. Mild cognitive impairment. N Engl J Med 2011;364(23):2227–34.
25. Marsh NV, Ludbrook MR, Gaffaney LC. Cognitive functioning following traumatic brain injury: a five-year follow-up. NeuroRehabilitation 2016;38(1):71–8.
26. Kaup AR, Peltz C, Kenney K, et al. Neuropsychological profile of lifetime traumatic brain injury in older veterans. J Int Neuropsychol Soc 2017;23(1):56–64.
27. Garcia CA, Tweedy JR, Blass JP. Underdiagnosis of cognitive impairment in a rehabilitation setting. J Am Geriatr Soc 1984;32(5):339–42. Available at: http://www.ncbi.nlm.nih.gov/pubmed/6715758. Accessed February 15, 2017.
28. Arciniegas DB, Frey KL, Newman J, et al. Evaluation and management of posttraumatic cognitive impairments. Psychiatr Ann 2010;40(11):540–52.
29. Cicerone KD, Langenbahn DM, Braden C, et al. Evidence-based cognitive rehabilitation: updated review of the literature from 2003 through 2008. Arch Phys Med Rehabil 2011;92(4):519–30.
30. Morris T, Gomes Osman J, Tormos Muñoz JM, et al. The role of physical exercise in cognitive recovery after traumatic brain injury: a systematic review. Restor Neurol Neurosci 2016;34(6):977–88.
31. Arciniegas DB, Silver JM. Pharmacotherapy of cognitive impairment. In: Zasler ND, Katz DI, Zafonte RD, editors. Brain injury medicine. 2nd edition. Principles and practice. 2013. p. 1215–26.
32. Barker-Collo S, Jones A, Jones K, et al. Prevalence, natural course and predictors of depression 1 year following traumatic brain injury from a population-based study in New Zealand. Brain Inj 2015;29(7–8):859–65.
33. Lyness JM, Cox C, Curry J, et al. Older age and the underreporting of depressive symptoms. J Am Geriatr Soc 1995;43(3):216–21. Available at: http://www.ncbi.nlm.nih.gov/pubmed/7884106. Accessed February 16, 2017.
34. Shahab S, Nicolici D-F, Tang A, et al. Depression predicts functional outcome in geriatric inpatient rehabilitation. Arch Phys Med Rehabil 2017;98(3):500–7.
35. Luck-Sikorski C, Stein J, Heilmann K, et al. Treatment preferences for depression in the elderly. Int Psychogeriatr 2017;29(3):389–98.
36. Graven C, Brock K, Hill KD, et al. First year after stroke. Stroke 2016;47(11):2820–7.
37. Plantier D, Luauté J, SOFMER Group. Drugs for behavior disorders after traumatic brain injury: systematic review and expert consensus leading to French recommendations for good practice. Ann Phys Rehabil Med 2016;59(1):42–57.
38. Arciniegas DB, Silver JM. Pharmacotherapy of neuropsychiatric disturbances. In: Zasler ND, Katz DI, Zafonte RD, editors. Brain injury medicine. 2nd edition. Principles and practice. 2013. p. 1227–44.
39. Rothenhäusler HB, Ehrentraut S, von Degenfeld G, et al. Treatment of depression with methylphenidate in patients difficult to wean from mechanical ventilation in the intensive care unit. J Clin Psychiatry 2000;61(10):750–5. Available at: http://www.ncbi.nlm.nih.gov/pubmed/11078036. Accessed February 17, 2017.
40. Schneider LS, Dagerman KS, Insel P. Risk of death with atypical antipsychotic drug treatment for dementia: meta-analysis of randomized placebo-controlled trials. JAMA 2005;294(15):1934–43.
41. Hartog LC, Winters AM, Roijen H, et al. The association between orthostatic hypotension and handgrip strength with successful rehabilitation in elderly hip fracture patients. Arch Phys Med Rehabil 2016. http://dx.doi.org/10.1016/j.apmr.2016.11.009.

42. Consensus statement on the definition of orthostatic hypotension, pure autonomic failure, and multiple system atrophy. J Neurol Sci 1996;144(1–2):218–9. Available at: http://www.ncbi.nlm.nih.gov/pubmed/8994128. Accessed February 17, 2017.

43. Swift CG, Iliffe S. Assessment and prevention of falls in older people - concise guidance. Clin Med (Lond) 2014;14(6):658–62.

44. Frewen J, Savva GM, Boyle G, et al. Cognitive performance in orthostatic hypotension: findings from a nationally representative sample. J Am Geriatr Soc 2014; 62(1):117–22. Available at: http://www.ncbi.nlm.nih.gov/pubmed/25180380. Accessed February 17, 2017.

45. Oishi E, Sakata S, Tsuchihashi T, et al. Orthostatic hypotension predicts a poor prognosis in elderly people with dementia. Intern Med 2016;55(15):1947–52.

46. Hoffman JM, Doctor JN, Chan L, et al. Potential impact of the new Medicare prospective payment system on reimbursement for traumatic brain injury inpatient rehabilitation. Arch Phys Med Rehabil 2003;84(8):1165–72.

47. Frankel JE, Marwitz JH, Cifu DX, et al. A follow-up study of older adults with traumatic brain injury: taking into account decreasing length of stay. Arch Phys Med Rehabil 2006;87(1):57–62.

48. Cifu DX, Kreutzer JS, Marwitz JH, et al. Functional outcomes of older adults with traumatic brain injury: a prospective, multicenter analysis. Arch Phys Med Rehabil 1996;77(9):883–8.

49. Cuthbert JP, Harrison-Felix C, Corrigan JD, et al. Epidemiology of Adults Receiving Acute Inpatient Rehabilitation for a Primary Diagnosis of traumatic brain injury in the United States. J Head Trauma Rehabil 2014;30(2):122–35.

50. Graham JE, Radice-Neumann DM, Reistetter TA, et al. Influence of sex and age on inpatient rehabilitation outcomes among older adults with traumatic brain injury. Arch Phys Med Rehabil 2010;91(1):43–50.

51. Vollmer DG, Torner JC, Jane JA, et al. Age and outcome following traumatic coma: why do older patients fare worse? J Neurosurg 1991;75:S37–49.

52. Thompson HJ, McCormick WC, Kagan SH. Traumatic brain injury in older adults: epidemiology, outcomes, and future implications. J Am Geriatr Soc 2006;54(10): 1590–5.

53. Mathias JL, Wheaton P. Contribution of brain or biological reserve and cognitive or neural reserve to outcome after TBI: a meta-analysis (prior to 2015). Neurosci Biobehav Rev 2015;55:573–93.

54. Peters ME. Traumatic brain injury (TBI) in older adults: aging with a TBI versus incident TBI in the aged. Int Psychogeriatr 2016;28(12):1931–4.

55. Eum RS, Brown AW, Watanabe TK, et al. Risk factors for institutionalization after traumatic brain injury inpatient rehabilitation. J Head Trauma Rehabil 2017;32(3): 158–67.

56. Marquez de la Plata CD, Hart T, Hammond FM, et al. Impact of Age on Long-Term Recovery From Traumatic Brain Injury. Arch Phys Med Rehabil 2008;89(5): 896–903. http://dx.doi.org/10.1016/j.apmr.2007.12.030.

57. Sendroy-Terrill M, Whiteneck GG, Brooks CA. Aging with traumatic brain injury: cross-sectional follow-up of people receiving inpatient rehabilitation over more than 3 decades. Arch Phys Med Rehabil 2010;91(3):489–97.

58. Hammond FM, Hart T, Bushnik T, et al. Change and predictors of change in communication, cognition, and social function between 1 and 5 years after traumatic brain injury. J Head Trauma Rehabil 2004;19(4):314–28.

59. Ritchie L, Wright-St Clair VA, Keogh J, et al. Community integration after traumatic brain injury: a systematic review of the clinical implications of measurement and service provision for older adults. Arch Phys Med Rehabil 2014;95(1):163–74.

60. Colantonio A, Ratcliff G, Chase S, et al. Long-term outcomes after moderate to severe traumatic brain injury. Disabil Rehabil 2004;26(5):253–61.
61. Dawn Senathi-Raja, Jennie Ponsford, Michael Schönberger. Association of age with long-term psychosocial outcome following traumatic brain injury. J Rehabil Med (Stiftelsen Rehabiliteringsinformation) 2009;41(8):666–73, 8p.
62. Testa JA, Malec JF, Moessner AM, et al. Outcome after traumatic brain injury: effects of aging on recovery. Arch Phys Med Rehabil 2005;86(9):1815–23.
63. Rapport LJ, Bryer RC, Hanks RA, et al. after traumatic brain injury. Arch Phys Med Rehabil 2008;89(5):922–30.
64. Whiteneck GG, Gerhart KA, Cusick CP. Identifying environmental factors that influence the outcomes of people with traumatic brain injury. J Head Trauma Rehabil 2004;19(3):191–204.
65. Kim H, Colantonio A. Effectiveness of rehabilitation in enhancing community integration after acute traumatic brain injury: a systematic review. Am J Occup Ther 2010;64(5):709–19.
66. Winkler D, Unsworth C, Sloan S. Factors that lead to successful community integration following severe traumatic brain injury. J Head Trauma Rehabil 2006; 21(1):8–21.
67. Deb S, Burns J. Neuropsychiatric consequences of traumatic brain injury: a comparison between two age groups. Brain Inj 2007;21(3):301–7.
68. Rapoport MJ, McCullagh S, Shammi P, et al. Cognitive Impairment Associated With Major Depression Following Mild and Moderate Traumatic Brain Injury. J Neuropsychiatry Clin Neurosci 2005;17(1):61–5.
69. Salat DH, Kaye JA, Janowsky JS. Prefrontal gray and white matter volumes in healthy aging and Alzheimer disease. Arch Neurol 1999;56:338–44.
70. Christodoulou C, DeLuca J, Ricker JH, et al. Functional magnetic resonance imaging of working memory impairment after traumatic brain injury. J Neurol Neurosurg Psychiatry 2001;71(2):161–8.
71. Hammond FM, Grattan KD, Sasser H, et al. Five years after traumatic brain injury: a study of individual outcomes and predictors of change in function. NeuroRehabilitation 2004;19(1):25–35.
72. Hammond FM, Grattan KD, Sasser H, et al. Long-term recovery course after traumatic brain injury: a comparison of the functional independence measure and disability rating scale. J Head Trauma Rehabil 2001;16(4):318–29.
73. Thomsen IV. Late outcome of very severe blunt head trauma: a 10-15 year second follow-up. J Neurol Neurosurg Psychiatry 1984;47(3):260–8.
74. Klein M, Houx PJ, Jolles J. Long-term persisting cognitive sequelae of traumatic brain injury and the effect of age. J Nerv Ment Dis 1996;184(8):459–67.
75. Ziebell JM, Rowe RK, Muccigrosso MM, et al. Aging with a traumatic brain injury: could behavioral morbidities and endocrine symptoms be influenced by microglial priming? Brain Behav Immun 2015;59:1–7.
76. Crane PK, Gibbons LE, Dams-O'Connor K, et al. Association of traumatic brain injury with late-life neurodegenerative conditions and neuropathologic findings. JAMA Neurol 2016;98104:7–14.
77. Wang H-K, Lin S-H, Sung P, et al. Population based study on patients with traumatic brain injury suggests increased risk of dementia. J Neurol Neurosurg Psychiatry 2012;83(11):1080–5.
78. Gardner RC, Burke JF, Nettiksimmons J, et al. Dementia risk after traumatic brain injury vs nonbrain trauma. JAMA Neurol 2014;71(12):1490.
79. Mendez MF, Paholpak P, Lin A, et al. Prevalence of traumatic brain injury in early versus late-onset Alzheimer's disease. J Alzheimers Dis 2015;47(4):985–93.

80. Li W, Risacher SL, McAllister TW, et al. Traumatic brain injury and age at onset of cognitive impairment in older adults. J Neurol 2016;263(7):1280–5.
81. Mortimer JA, Van Duijn CM, Chandra L, et al. Head trauma as a risk factor for Alzheimer's disease: a collaborative reanalysis of case control studies. Int J Epidemiol 1991;20(Suppl_2):25–35.
82. Roberts GW, Gentleman SM, Lynch A, et al. Beta amyloid protein deposition in the brain after severe head injury: implications for the pathogenesis of Alzheimer's disease. J Neurol Neurosurg Psychiatry 1994;57(4):419–25.
83. Horsburgh K, McCarron MO, White F, et al. The role of apolipoprotein E in Alzheimer's disease, acute brain injury and cerebrovascular disease: evidence of common mechanisms and utility of animal models. Neurobiol Aging 2000; 21(2):245–55.
84. Nicoll JA, Roberts GW, Graham DI. Apolipoprotein E epsilon 4 allele is associated with deposition of amyloid beta-protein following head injury. Nat Med 1995;1(2): 135–7.
85. Jordan D, Relkin NR, Ravdin LD, et al. Apolipoprotein chronic traumatic brain injury in boxing. JAMA 1997;278:136–40.
86. Crawford FC, Vanderploeg RD, Freeman MJ, et al. APOE genotype influences acquisition and recall following traumatic brain injury. Neurology 2002;58(7): 1115–8.
87. Lichtman SW, Seliger G, Tycko B, et al. Apolipoprotein E and functional recovery from brain injury following postacute rehabilitation. Neurology 2000;55(10): 1536–9.
88. Friedman G, Froom P, Sazbon L, et al. Apolipoprotein E-epsilon4 genotype predicts a poor outcome in survivors of traumatic brain injury. Neurology 1999;52(2): 244–8.
89. Brooks JC, Shavelle RM, Strauss DJ, et al. Long-term survival after traumatic brain injury part II: life expectancy. Arch Phys Med Rehabil 2015;96(6):1000–5.
90. Harrison-Felix C, Pretz C, Hammond FM, et al. Life expectancy after inpatient rehabilitation for traumatic brain injury in the United States. J Neurotrauma 2015;32(23):1893–901.
91. Harrison-Felix C, Kolakowsky-Hayner SA, Hammond FM, et al. Mortality after surviving traumatic brain injury. J Head Trauma Rehabil 2012;27(6):E45–56.

UNITED STATES POSTAL SERVICE ® **Statement of Ownership, Management, and Circulation (All Periodicals Publications Except Requester Publications)**

1. Publication Title	2. Publication Number	3. Filing Date
PHYSICAL MEDICINE AND REHABILITATION CLINICS OF NORTH AMERICA	009 – 243	9/18/2017

4. Issue Frequency	5. Number of Issues Published Annually	6. Annual Subscription Price
FEB, MAY, AUG, NOV	4	$288.00

7. Complete Mailing Address of Known Office of Publication (Not printer) (Street, city, county, state, and ZIP+4®)

ELSEVIER INC.
230 Park Avenue, Suite 800
New York, NY 10169

Contact Person
STEPHEN R. BUSHING
Telephone (Include area code)
215-239-3688

8. Complete Mailing Address of Headquarters or General Business Office of Publisher (Not printer)

ELSEVIER INC.
230 Park Avenue, Suite 800
New York, NY 10169

9. Full Names and Complete Mailing Addresses of Publisher, Editor, and Managing Editor (Do not leave blank)

Publisher (Name and complete mailing address)

ADRIANNE BRIGIDO, ELSEVIER INC.
1600 JOHN F KENNEDY BLVD. SUITE 1800
PHILADELPHIA, PA 19103-2899

Editor (Name and complete mailing address)

LAUREN BOYLE, ELSEVIER INC.
1600 JOHN F KENNEDY BLVD. SUITE 1800
PHILADELPHIA, PA 19103-2899

Managing Editor (Name and complete mailing address)

PATRICK MANLEY, ELSEVIER INC.
1600 JOHN F KENNEDY BLVD. SUITE 1800
PHILADELPHIA, PA 19103-2899

10. Owner (Do not leave blank. If the publication is owned by a corporation, give the name and address of the corporation immediately followed by the names and addresses of all stockholders owning or holding 1 percent or more of the total amount of stock. If not owned by a corporation, give the names and addresses of the individual owners. If owned by a partnership or other unincorporated firm, give its name and address as well as those of each individual owner. If the publication is published by a nonprofit organization, give its name and address.)

Full Name	Complete Mailing Address
WHOLLY OWNED SUBSIDIARY OF REED/ELSEVIER, US HOLDINGS	1600 JOHN F KENNEDY BLVD. SUITE 1800 PHILADELPHIA, PA 19103-2899

11. Known Bondholders, Mortgagees, and Other Security Holders Owning or Holding 1 Percent or More of Total Amount of Bonds, Mortgages, or Other Securities. If none, check box ▶ ☐ None

Full Name	Complete Mailing Address
N/A	

12. Tax Status (For completion by nonprofit organizations authorized to mail at nonprofit rates) (Check one)
The purpose, function, and nonprofit status of this organization and the exempt status for federal income tax purposes:
☒ Has Not Changed During Preceding 12 Months
☐ Has Changed During Preceding 12 Months (Publisher must submit explanation of change with this statement)

13. Publication Title	14. Issue Date for Circulation Data Below
PHYSICAL MEDICINE AND REHABILITATION CLINICS OF NORTH AMERICA	AUGUST 2017

15. Extent and Nature of Circulation		Average No. Copies Each Issue During Preceding 12 Months	No. Copies of Single Issue Published Nearest to Filing Date
a. Total Number of Copies (Net press run)		325	283
b. Paid Circulation (By Mail and Outside the Mail)	(1) Mailed Outside-County Paid Subscriptions Stated on PS Form 3541 (Include paid distribution above nominal rate, advertiser's proof copies, and exchange copies)	166	145
	(2) Mailed In-County Paid Subscriptions Stated on PS Form 3541 (Include paid distribution above nominal rate, advertiser's proof copies, and exchange copies)	0	0
	(3) Paid Distribution Outside the Mails Including Sales Through Dealers and Carriers, Street Vendors, Counter Sales, and Other Paid Distribution Outside USPS®	71	67
	(4) Paid Distribution by Other Classes of Mail Through the USPS (e.g. First-Class Mail®)	0	0
c. Total Paid Distribution (Sum of 15b (1), (2), (3), and (4))		237	212
d. Free or Nominal Rate Distribution (By Mail and Outside the Mail)	(1) Free or Nominal Rate Outside-County Copies included on PS Form 3541	40	71
	(2) Free or Nominal Rate In-County Copies included on PS Form 3541	0	0
	(3) Free or Nominal Rate Copies Mailed at Other Classes Through the USPS (e.g. First-Class Mail)	0	0
	(4) Free or Nominal Rate Distribution Outside the Mail (Carriers or other means)	0	0
e. Total Free or Nominal Rate Distribution (Sum of 15d (1), (2), (3) and (4))		40	71
f. Total Distribution (Sum of 15c and 15e)		277	283
g. Copies not Distributed (See Instructions to Publishers #4 (page #3))		48	0
h. Total (Sum of 15f and g)		325	283
i. Percent Paid (15c divided by 15f times 100)		85.56%	74.91%

* If you are claiming electronic copies, go to line 16 on page 3. If you are not claiming electronic copies, skip to line 17 on page 3.

16. Electronic Copy Circulation		Average No. Copies Each Issue During Preceding 12 Months	No. Copies of Single Issue Published Nearest to Filing Date
a. Paid Electronic Copies	▶	0	0
b. Total Paid Print Copies (Line 15c) + Paid Electronic Copies (Line 16a)	▶	237	212
c. Total Print Distribution (Line 15f) + Paid Electronic Copies (Line 16a)	▶	277	283
d. Percent Paid (Both Print & Electronic Copies) (16b divided by 16c × 100)	▶	85.56%	74.91%

☒ I certify that 50% of all my distributed copies (electronic and print) are paid above a nominal price.

17. Publication of Statement of Ownership
☒ If the publication is a general publication, publication of this statement is required. Will be printed ☐ Publication not required.
in the NOVEMBER 2017 issue of this publication.

18. Signature and Title of Editor, Publisher, Business Manager, or Owner

STEPHEN R. BUSHING - INVENTORY DISTRIBUTION CONTROL MANAGER

Date 9/18/2017

I certify that all information furnished on this form is true and complete. I understand that anyone who furnishes false or misleading information on this form or who omits material or information requested on the form may be subject to criminal sanctions (including fines and imprisonment) and/or civil sanctions (including civil penalties).

PS Form **3526**, July 2014 (Page 1 of 4 (see instructions page 4)) PSN: 7530-01-000-9931 PRIVACY NOTICE: See our privacy policy on www.usps.com.

PS Form **3526**, July 2014 (Page 2 of 4) PRIVACY NOTICE: See our privacy policy on www.usps.com.

Printed and bound by CPI Group (UK) Ltd, Croydon, CR0 4YY

03/10/2024

01040390-0020